# *Winning the Battle Against Cancer:*

## *They said I was going to die… but, I didn't*

### *Elaine Hulliberger*

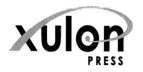

XULON PRESS

*Winning the Battle Against Cancer:*
*They said I was going to die...but, I didn't*
by Elaine Hulliberger

Printed in the United States of America

ISBN 978-1-60647-056-5

First Edition

www.xulonpress.com

# About The Author

Elaine had what most of us want, a good family, a good job, and good health. Then, her husband dropped dead at her feet. Three months later she finds she had terminal cancer, and she lost her lively-hood. Doctors told her she has less than 2 months to live. She's devastated and broken. Then she found a way to turn her life around.

It's her story. It's a story of a woman who looks up at seemingly insurmountable mountains of grief, then turned it into faith, courage, and a road back to life. She shows you that cancer can be cured, not merely put into remission. She'll show you that you have choices and options, and that you can retain your dignity and self-worth after being dismissed by the medical world. She'll show you a more humane world of cancer treatments that can actually cure your cancer. Elaine won her ***Battle Against Cancer***, and so can you.

The author can be reached at hully@netonecom.net

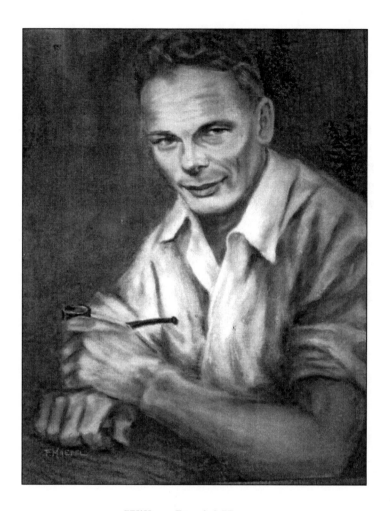

**Wilbur Daniel Hearn**
**February 1911 – January 1987**
**Memorial Dedication**

This book is a memorial dedication to my dad, the first and best man I ever depended on, and the kindest dad a little girl could hope for. Without his guidance I wouldn't be who I am today. He taught me to respect others. He taught me work ethics, and he taught me how to be strong. He answered any question I asked him, and through most of the questions; he kept a straight face. He was a man of honor. When he gave his word, they were words you could count on.

One look from him was all it took for me to know whether I was right in what I was doing, or wrong. If the latter was the case, he gave me the chance to correct my error to the best of my abilities. Otherwise, he would 'help' me understand a better way. His help let me know that I had better actions and thoughts to give. He let me know that, whatever I did, he would always be there for me. And...he was. I valued his friendship, he always stood by me, and his teachings were gentle. I am proud of the heritage he gave to me, and I am grateful that my ways are his ways. He will always be the first man in my life, and I will always be his loving daughter.

I love you Dad...

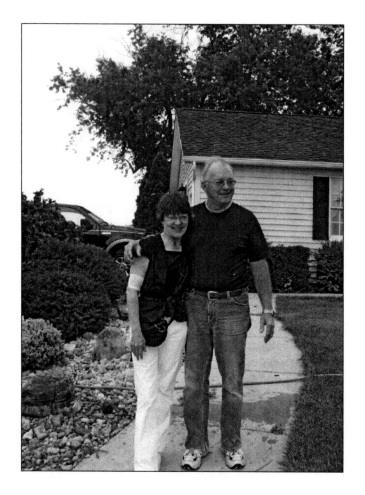

**A special dedication to:
Duane L. Hearn
My brother, my friend**

My brother doesn't look upon himself as a great man, although he is. He doesn't consider what he did for me as 'out of the ordinary', but I do. See how he has his arm positioned in the picture above? His heart, his protection, and his love for me are positioned in just that way.

We are both strong people, because we were raised to believe we should be, therefore we could be strong. We love each other because we respect each other. But, I am alive today because he protected me, because he believed in me, and because he wanted, and needed to be a part of my recovery. Without him...I had no one close enough to help me. Without him I wouldn't be here. But, I...am...here!

He is the storybook definition of "brother". He has always been my hero, and he always will be. He made me laugh when I didn't think I could. He put me under his protective arm when I had no one else. He put up with my moodiness, and he was gracious about it. He toughened up my resolve to collide with cancer when I didn't think I could, and he stood by me in the absolute until I was well. He is my brother... and I am loved. He is my brother...and I am alive.

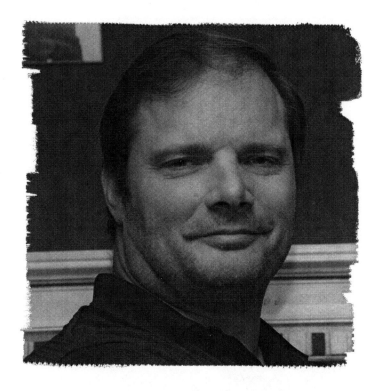

**Randall A Leutz**
**My son...**

When things were dark, and no light found
When life was changed, and fears abound
You were there...
The battle seemed an endless chore
When life, it felt, would be no more...
You were there...
Our roles reversed, you took the lead,
Your strength and kindness filled my need...
You were there...

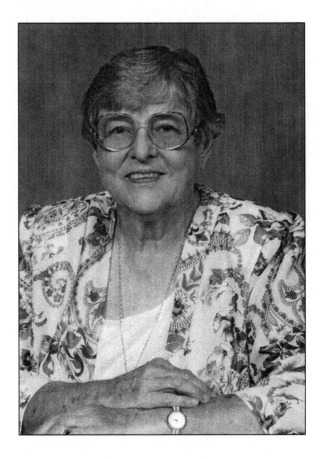

# SPECIAL ACKNOWLEDGEMENT

My mom...she was, and remains, so very supportive. She must have laid in bed at night thinking up things to say to me, and things to do for me that she thought would help me through. I was so scared in the beginning, I was desperately lonely, and I was in need of her support; the sort of support that only a mom can give. She helped me more than she will ever know. I think of women who may not have a mom to lean on when their life turns inside out. How grateful I am that she was there for me. God bless you mom. I love you.

## A Special Tribute to Dale
## Written by Shawn Maxwell

# Dale

I never told you what you were to me
-   -The person I looked up to
    -My advisor
    -My teacher
It just wasn't manly to tell you that...

I never told you what I saw in you
-   -Pride
    -Honor
    -Happiness

I never told you what you have done
for me
-   - You gave me a different look
    on life
    -You gave me courage
    - You gave me strength

It just wasn't manly to tell you that...

I never told you how much you have
helped me
-   -A pat on the back when I
    was feeling down
    -A quick laugh when I
    was hurting
    -A word of advice when I
    was making a mistake
It wasn't manly to tell you that...

I never told you how much you
made me laugh
-   -A smart-ass comment
    -The way you would
    curse yourself when you did
    something wrong
    -The way it took an hour
    for you to answer a question
    (because you were thinking
    about it)
It just wasn't manly to tell you that...

I never told you how I felt
about you
-   -You're my hero
    -You're my best friend
    -I love you...
    In a manly sort of way...

*Love*

*Shaun*

# Acknowledgements

I want to give special thanks to Alex Wolf for his timely help. We got to know one another because his wife was suffering with cancer. His heart and soul was filled with grief, and he was looking for some answers. But, in all of his personal suffering over his wife, he let me borrow his beautiful daughter for my book cover. Thank you Alex... from the bottom of my heart.

A large dose of thanks go to John Nelson's Studios in Cadillac, MI. I asked him to do the photo you see on the back of this book. I looked at it as a mission. He had to make me look good. All the chemotherapy, stress, and 'age' would present him with a challenge. It's apparent that he was up to the challenge, because I think it turned out great. When I told him what the photo was for, he donated his efforts, his talents, time, and his considerable knowledge to my effort. Thank you so very much John.

John can be reached at:
John Nelson Photography
110 N. Mitchell St
Cadillac, MI 49601

Dr. Philip Philip and Karmanos Cancer Treatment Center in Detroit, Michigan deserves acknowledgement and my grateful thanks for giving me the chance to fight for my life when I didn't think anyone could or would. Had it not been for Dr. Philip's initial decision to try to help me...I wouldn't be here today. I see his face yet today when I close my eyes in prayer.

Dr. J. Hamamdjian of Southfield, Michigan is one of the kindest, most thorough, and most knowledgeable doctors I've ever known. He explained everything to me in layman-friendly terms; terms that even I could understand, and his initial reaction was simply concern. How good that felt at the time. He didn't look at me and see hopelessness...even in the beginning. All he cared about was that he could help me get through this horrible cancer. And he did just that.

There are no words to express what my friends meant to me through all of the dark days. Their support, love, kindness, thoughtfulness, and so much more just blow my mind. They are awesome people who deserve more words of thanks than I can ever say. I'll just say this, "I will always love all of you, I am way past grateful, and I will never ever forget". I will never forget your words, your kindness, your concern, and your love. I will always try to live up to your friendship. I will never forget...

Most of all, "Thank you Jesus". You helped me through. You showed me Your love for me. You whispered hope in my ear. You gave my life back to me. I will spend the rest of my life trying to be what You want me to be. If there is any one thing that brings me to tears yet today...it's Your love. Because of You...I am never alone. Because of Your love, I am alive.

# Foreword

When my life began I was totally dependent on someone else to keep me alive. After a while, I learned to do that on my own. Then, I was taught what to think, how to feel, and what to do. Parents, schools, television, friends, and relatives all played a role in developing my personality. I am the product of my childhood. I have become what I saw back then, and what I was taught.

When I became an adult I did what my parents did. I lived my life directed mostly by my childhood memories. There's nothing unusual about any of this. We all do it to some degree or other. We do the best we can with what we've been dealt. One day turns into the next, and the New Year follows the old. Life becomes almost predictable, doesn't it?

Then, you're hit right between the eyes with the mother lode. You have been diagnosed with a terrible disease, and you're told there is nothing that can be done. You're told you are going to die. *What do you do?*

You can believe what your doctor(s) tell you, and do what they tell you to do. You can get your affairs in order. You can prepare yourself, as best you can, for your death. You can, and will; get angry, cry, and feel unimaginable fear. You may bargain with God. You'll feel emotions that are familiar, and emotions that you didn't know existed. When you've done all you know how to do, you're left to face the reality of your own death. From that point on your life is in your hands.

The first question you'll have to answer is; am I going to give up? Or, are you going to become an active part in what it takes to cure your disease? Can you muster enough courage, strength, and faith to fight to live? Sure you can! But, this is one of those few times in your life when the decisions you make rests entirely with you.

You're facing off with the monster that everyone fears. How do you make the monster back off? You draw that line in the sand. You dig deep down in your very soul for the strength you need to believe in tomorrow. You fight! No one can make you fight, but no one can talk you out of the battle it you don't allow it. You believe in victory! You believe in...you.

What if you give everything to the battle, but loose in the end. What if you don't?

What if the doctors are right about you? What if they're wrong?

How do you fight it? I can only tell you how I fought. You will wage your own war. You'll do things your own way. But, you'll do it. You'll find a way.

I may not know you, but you can bet that I'm on your side. I may not know your name, but I can pray for you just the same. You'll get to know me by reading my story. *I know you because of my story.*

# A Personal Message to You

Before I begin my story I want you to know that, you as a cancer patient, can have a say in your treatments. I'm not suggesting that you become your own doctor. What I am suggesting is this:

If you feel uncomfortable with your treatment, then ask questions. If your doctor can't, or won't answer your questions, then find one who can or will. If you're being treated with less than respect, find another doctor who will give you his emotional support along with his medical support.

Any good doctor is aware of how important good emotions are to the recovery process. His job should be to help you get well in any way he can. That includes giving you as much hope and compassion as he would expect under the same circumstances. I'm not suggesting doctors are gods or infallible, but I am suggesting there is more to cancer than chemotherapy, radiation, surgery and fees. When doctors forget compassion they've lost the ability to fully treat and heal.

The same is true when they can't, or won't, consider non-toxic products or natural supplements. Natural/non-toxic supplements can play a very large role in your cancer treatments. Unfortunately, you will have to use your own initiative to learn about them. *But...do learn.* My point is this: Don't let your illness progress and your health deteriorate because of your doctor's belief that conventional medicine is the only way to control cancer. *It surely is not.* And, certainly, don't let his inability to believe in you be the deciding factor in whether you will live or die.

I believe that the patient should be given the ***choice*** to fight for his or her own life; even when the doctor may not believe there is any hope in non-toxic products, or that conventional medicine won't help. Certainly, doctors see a lot. Because of that, their advice is a result of their experience. I believe it is that experience that tells them when it's time to give up on the disease and the patient. Many of them feel the nightmare that conventional treatments cause isn't worth losing what quality of life the patient has left. The same dyer outcome is predicted because they're absolutely sure there are no non-toxic products that can work.

Consequently, they believe there are no choices left. If you believe what they say about all of this...if you truly believe you can't win...you probably won't. If you allow belief in yourself, if you fight when you don't think you can...if you fight to win, than you probably will. You may or may not agree. The point is that it isn't the doctor's decision to make. It's yours.

What if the doctors are wrong about you? What if you're the exception to the rule? What if there is something inside you, just one tiny thing that the doctor can't see that could see you through? Even if you don't have a clear understanding of what that *something* is that's inside you; that *something* is ready to change the odds in your favor. I don't know what to call it either... but, I know it's there. I had it...we all have it, and you have it! You have it! What if you can beat this cancer against all odds? It happens...it really can happen.

Remember this; your *willingness* to fight will give you the *ability* to fight.

Don't let doctors take away your right to fight. Don't lose hope in your recovery because a doctor may not know what tremendous strength you have in your soul. Don't let them give your life away because they don't understand, or believe, that there are less invasive ways to kill your cancer. I know you have what it takes, and <u>so do you.</u>

So, if you have cancer...don't give in to it – collide with it! If you have a loved one with cancer, then help them dig in for the fight of their life. Be their champion when they need one. They can't win the war if they don't face the battle. Join them. Help them. You'll find a tremendous amount of love there. I'm still here because I chose to fight when all the odds were against me, and I found loving friends and family members who were willing to help me. God bless them... every one.

None of the doctors I spoke with in the beginning gave me the choice to fight, and none of them explained why they had made that decision. I was too stunned and confused to ask the right questions, and they didn't offer answers. I didn't know where the cancer was, and had no idea how far it had advanced. In the beginning, you see, all they were basing their diagnosis on was the single original biopsy and a blood test.

There are other diagnostic tools that should have been used before I made reservations for my own funeral. So, the first stage of the struggle was finding someone who would allow me the right to the battle, and to help me fight it. I felt that if nothing could be done, then so be it. However, if something could be done, than I wanted the chance to try. I wanted to know I had done everything I could do as I took my last breath. And, that's just what happened. The 'everything' I chose to, or learned to do was enough to see me through, and that's just the way it ended up.

Read on. I'm the proof you're looking for. God is your hope, your wits are your resource, and your health is on its way back to you. B.E.L.I.E.V.E!

# Winning The
# Battle Against Cancer

## They said I was going to die...but, I didn't

The will of God won't lead you where the love of God
won't protect you.

# Where it All Began

On August 7, 2005 my husband walked up to me in a restaurant and fell dead at my feet. There was no warning, he hadn't been ill, so all that was left was shock and disbelief. There are no words to explain what I felt or what followed. Nothing felt real, and yet what I did feel was totally and indescribably devastating. There was his funeral, and there were days and nights filled with grief. All of a sudden I was alone, and life meant little to me.

Dale and I were married in February of 1991. I married him because he was a quiet man with an unexpected sense of humor. He made me laugh. He was as honest as a person could be. I trusted him. He was innovative. I needed him. He showed me that he was proud of me. I married Dale because I loved him.

Dale had a supervisory position in the injection-molding department of the factory where we worked. I was an inspector, then the liaison for the new jobs that came into the plant, then went back to inspection. We were happy with one another, and reasonably happy with our work.

With Dale's blessings, I quit my job in 1996 to begin a commercial embroidery business. Three years later I added dye-sublimation to the processes.

The business grew until I was earning as much in the business as I made while working in the factory. The difference was that I truly loved what I was doing, although many times it got pretty hectic. When I had large orders that I couldn't get finished on time and without help, Dale would pitch in after he got home from work. It was a lot of work but we enjoyed it, and we began to wish that Dale could afford to quit his supervisory job to help build and run the business.

## Be careful what you pray for...

After working for that company for 34 years, he was downsized. No warning, no benefits, and no explanation. When I saw him drive in our parking lot at 11:30 that morning, I knew what had happened. When he came through the door the only thing he said was, "All I need is your support". His facial expression said the rest.

He received nothing on his last day of work except two months of regular pay, six weeks of unemployment, and no benefits of any kind. That day our future was totally changed, and everything seemed to screech to a complete standstill.

I can't imagine what he must have felt that day, as I'd never had to face that sort of complete dismissal. At that moment, I think, the past 34 years seemed to be important to no one but himself. However, somewhere in all of his immediate emotions I could sense his resolve and strength begin to rise to the surface. We decided to make this work in our favor.

The first thing we did was separate the two processes in our business. I kept the embroidery, and Dale took over the dye sublimation. He took the dye sublimation and made it his own, and began to build it from his heart. He and his business literally bloomed. You could tell he was finding satisfaction in what he was doing for the first time in his working life. It became obvious that the real Dale had been waiting patiently for his time to earn his living by his wits and talents. Watching him learn to live as he was meant to live is one of my valued memories. It was a gift that God gave Dale. We had fifteen months together being what we had never been before, doing what we loved to do, and getting to know our real selves. It was a most enjoyable time for us.

Then, without warning, it was all over. He was gone in seconds that seemed like an eternity. God put His hand on both of us in that instant. He took Dale home, and began teaching me how to get through the loss. It's good that God had confidence in my recovery, because I did not.

Grieving is something that takes on a life of its own and is all consuming. It isn't something that is easy to tell about, as most of it is done in a sort of numbed fog-like state. There were whole days that I don't remember much about. I never quite knew what to do next. I didn't know what to say to anyone. One minute I seemed okay, and the next minute I was in that empty void. I knew I had to live, but I didn't know how I would do that. I wanted to love and to be loved, but I had lost it. I was a certifiable mess.

I did the only thing I knew to do. I prayed that God would give me the strength, courage, and faith I so desperately needed. I wasn't especially rational at that particular moment, so I don't believe I expected the prayer would be answered. But, It was. I don't know where I would be right now if the prayer hadn't been offered and answered. He gave me an abundance of strength, a ton of courage, and a bushel of faith. It was a good thing, as I was headed for the fight of my life, and the outcome was less than favorable.

I went through the next three months waking from sleep, floating through days that are difficult to remember, and then at night fighting for sleep again. I went to the cemetery hoping to feel closer to him, but he wasn't there. I would straighten his flowers, stand there waiting for something to happen, then when it didn't I'd go home to begin it all over again.

Sometimes I would eat. Most of the time I wasn't hungry so I lost some weight. I didn't want to go anywhere. I didn't want to do anything. I didn't know what to do. It was all part of the grieving process, the beginning of a different kind of life, and I didn't like it at all. But, who does?

# The Cancer

Ihad found a lump on the back of my right shoulder earlier
that spring. Even though cancer was found in my left breast
less than 30 days after Dale and I were married back in 1991,
I was sure this lump was an injury caused from throwing
a ball for our dog. After all, it had been 14 years since the
breast cancer and radiation. Besides, I'd had trouble with
shoulder injuries in the past from working in the factory. It
was an injury. It would go away in time.

However, by November of 2005 the lump was still promi-
nent and began to feel uncomfortable now and then. I wanted
to get it taken care of and so finally went to the doctor for an
examination. My family doctor told me what she thought it
could be, but I was sure it was merely an injury. However,
she arranged an appointment with an area surgeon for the
first appointment date he had open. I left her office believing
I had no cancer and would be just fine. I didn't feel particu-
larly ditzy that day, but apparently…I was.

I kept the appointment, and was examined by the young
surgeon. He suggested that I have the lump removed and
biopsied, although cancer didn't typically present itself in
the soft tissue of the body. He thought it was better to be

safe than sorry. I agreed that the operation was probably a good idea. I thought he would remove the lump, the injury would be corrected, and that would be that. So my surgery was scheduled for the day before Thanksgiving.

All the pre-op tests were taken care of before the day of surgery arrived. So, all I had to do when I got to the hospital was put on a hospital gown and hop on the gurney. And there I sat…waiting.

Okay, I thought…where's the drugs? I want to go to sleep. But, luck wasn't with me. I was taken to a hallway in the surgical unit, and left there for over an hour…without a blanket. Therefore, I had to be very careful about the back of my hospital gown. It was so big, though, that I could wrap it around my body a couple of times and still have enough 'gown' left for another wrap or two. Why do they make those things so big? I'm sure you've noticed that modesty isn't a real big concern in a hospital, but it was for me. I should have brought my PJ's. There was another patient on the other side of the hallway that I chitchatted with to pass the time. He had a blanket. That didn't help my mood.

I've never been accused of being a patient person, and this was getting on the last nerve I had left. I began to wonder where my clothes were. I wanted to go home. I was contemplating leaving when they came to get me. There was to be no escape.

Any surgery I'd had in the past was done well after a pre-op shot, the sort of shot that brings on sleep. But, there I was… lying on the surgery table...in surgery…and I was still wide-awake. I thought how this wasn't a good thing. I didn't think they were going to do the biopsy with me yelling and screaming, but no one seemed concerned about the fact that I was still awake, and way too alert, but me. Finally, I was given an IV with the anesthesiologist standing at the front of the table. I was in an irritable mood when I asked him if I was going to get sleepy any time soon. He said, "Good bye", and that's the last I remember. We must have parted as friends, because…I woke up…

I remember the day I drove to the doctor's office for my scheduled post-op examination. Given it was November in Michigan the weather wasn't bad at all, and, where I live traffic isn't an issue. I just breezed along listening to the radio and wondered to myself what I would do about Christmas. I didn't want to spend it with a family, and I didn't want to spend it alone. Not many choices left, is there. Oh well, I would think of something.

As always, I was early for the appointment, so I grabbed a magazine and waited. After a bit I was called to the examination room, sat on the exam table, and waited for the doctor. When he came in, I gave him a greeting then asked him what the biopsy showed. He said we would get to that in a minute. He chitchatted for as long as he could before he gave me the news. The lump had been removed successfully. He said, it was biopsied, and was found to be the size of a golf ball; and it was malignant.

I was shocked that I could have been so wrong about such a serious thing. When he told me about the cancer I was as stunned as anyone would have been. As I listened to him talk time seemed to stop for an instant, and I slipped into another world that was not familiar to me. It was a world with a door that slammed shut. A world that wouldn't let me back in to the one I had always known. I knew that nothing would ever be the same again. One second ago I was me, but I wasn't me anymore.

When the diagnosis hit home fear flooded my every fiber. Cancer began its emotional destruction at that very moment. I realized that the catastrophe that happened only to other people was now happening to me. The only thing I wanted to do was to go find Dale. I wanted to be where he was. I wanted to feel safe again. I didn't realize at the time just how close I was to having that wish granted.

The surgeon gave me all the information he had, however more detailed information would have to come from an oncologist. The surgeon suggested I contact my family doctor to have an appointment set up with an oncologist. He told me how sorry he was to have to give me the news. He had done all he could do, and so, my visit with him was over. When I left his office I didn't know where the cancer was, or if it had metastasized. All I knew was that I had cancer... again.

I didn't know what to think. How do others take news like this? What should I do now...what should I do first? Who should I tell, and when I tell them, what should I say? Where does a person start, and how am I going to get through this alone? It had only been three months since Dale's death, and I wanted him with me. I don't know if I'd ever felt more alone. I was so wrapped up in myself that I didn't even think of God. How could this happen? Wasn't one tragedy at a time enough? What's up with life anyway?

As I drove home I remember thinking that I was about to find out what I was made of. It's curious to me why that particular thought should have come to mind, but it did. I had no clue what was ahead for me, but I knew I had to get some sort of treatment begun, and the sooner the better. The war was declared and it was time to fight or die.

I made another appointment with my family doctor and asked her to set up an appointment with a good oncologist. She said she would set the appointment with an oncologist who was affiliated with the same medical facility that she worked with. Within a day or two an appointment was set with my first oncologist for the end of December. As I waited out the month for the appointment date to roll around I tried, with a fair amount of success, to dismiss the cancer issue. I didn't know what was ahead, and really didn't want to dwell on it. The business end of the world of cancer hadn't opened up to me yet. However, I was about to get an education...call it a crash course in how a bad situation can go downhill in a hurry.

I'm sure that most people believe the medical community will take a patient's cancer as seriously as the patient and their family does. You would expect to get a diagnosis and treatment begun as quickly as possible. I know I did. But, guess what...I couldn't have been more mistaken. I'm thankful that I didn't know then what was coming my way. Had I known, I'm afraid, I would have been tempted to give it all up right then and there. But...only tempted.

## Welcome to Reality

I kept the appointment with my first oncologist in December. I was understandably nervous and waiting in the examination room when the doctor came in. He introduced himself then asked me to get on the table behind the curtain. He wanted to do an examination. *...I obeyed...*

Doctors have examined me many times, for one reason or the other, during my life. It's always been a little uncomfortable I guess, but I've always been aware of how it was done. Maybe the doctor is feeling for a broken bone, or maybe it's something more serious that he's looking for. But, all times, it's as though he was listening through his touch. His mind hears what his touch is telling him. He is tuned in somehow, and he is quiet until that part of the examination is over. However, this examination was different. It was more of a cop-like frisk than an examination. It was as though this examination was unnecessary. He acted as though he knew what was there, where it was, and he knew the examination was a waste of time. It was expected, and it was done. End of story.

I expected some compassion, or maybe a little concern. What I felt was violated. I got down from the table, and we took a seat on the other side of the curtain. I should have left the building and kept going until I got home, but I was new to this sort of thing, and I was scared. I needed help.

I just stared at him when I found him to be void of anything that could be construed as a bedside manner. I was confused by his impatient approach, and he was rather rude. There was no kindness in his voice, and he was clinically cool in his character. He acted as though he had done this a million times before, and he was late for his next patient. I wanted my cancer to matter to him. I wanted 'me' to matter to him. But, neither seemed to matter at all.

I admit his attitude took my mind off my cancer for a moment as I tried to figure out where he came from, and what made him so cynical. Other than I felt he was a veri-fiable jerk, I couldn't quite figure where he attained such an impatient and sanctimonious attitude. However, I was slammed back to my own reality with his diagnosis.

Please remember that, so far, I hadn't had any sort of diagnostic scan, only the biopsy and a blood test. He gave me his diagnosis like he was recounting a sitcom rerun that he had very little interest in, a rerun that he had seen many times before. Simply put...it was my turn with cancer. It was merely my turn.

He said I had lymphoma, which was an incomplete diag-nosis at best. Had he treated me with the medications that were developed for lymphoma, would they have done any good? No. I'm sure his diagnosis and subsequent treatment would have been my undoing. The thing is, he didn't have enough information to diagnosis my condition at all, and it didn't seem to be an issue with him. I define that as unadul-terated arrogance. Knowing what I know now, I call that a "death sentence".

I remember wondering where he had gotten the informa-tion he used for the diagnosis. I knew the tests I'd had (the biopsy and a blood test), and thought there should be a little more information to consider before a diagnosis was given.

At the time, I was too stunned to ask and he didn't offer an explanation. It's just as well I guess, as I was past upset and headed for freaked out. I desperately needed some sort of hope to hold on to, but he gave me none at all. Any positive thought would have done wonders. A little warmth or compassion would have been enough for that day. However, he wasn't the sort to have thought of compassion, so I was left greatly lacking.

His prognosis was sure death for me. I could fight, he said, but it would always come back. The cancer *might* be put into remission, but it would only come back. I was going to die. Where is the compassion in that? Why couldn't he have said something like, "Your cancer is late stage and is tough, but let's try"? Please, tell me how a patient can fight without hope?

I asked him how long I had to live, and he simply said he had no idea. He could have said there was no way to really know, or, let's do some testing before we make that sort of judgment, or I'm sorry, Elaine, I just don't know. Nope. "I have no idea" was all I got from him.

I began to feel desperation set in, so I asked him about natural supplements that have the ability to kill cancer cells. Big mistake! I could tell he was upset with the question when he ignorantly and arrogantly answered, "They don't work!"

It's intriguing, isn't it, how a doctor can look down on you even when you're at eye level with one another? But, it's when his eyes glaze over that you know you've insulted his intelligences. As my question wafted into his ears it was blazingly clear to me that I was surely viewed as an uneducated bore with the intelligences of a limp pickle. He made me feel… well… stupid. And so…I bristled. I asked him why they didn't work, which seemed to me a reasonable question. Although I was getting pretty angry by now, *I couldn't wait for his answer.*

Although it wouldn't have cost him a nickel to either answer, or ignore the question he did neither. His voice went up and octave and he said, "Because they don't!" That's when I learned that one needs to be very careful what one asks an oncologist. You mustn't bother them with questions. I felt like running away, or insulting him back. I did neither.

He readied himself to leave the examination room with a parting comment that implied I should keep a good attitude. I guess I don't know why he tossed that in. It didn't seem to me that he cared much what happened to me one way or the other. That isn't bitterness speaking its mind. That's just the way it was.

As you can see some oncologists seem to be a little more thin-skinned about natural supplements and than others. So, just in case you contemplate asking an oncologist about natural supplements...you may want to reconsider, or brace yourself. Most of them will just ignore those types of questions. Some may even discuss supplements (let me know if you find one). Others, like this oncologist, will let you know you've scuffed the sandals they wear when they walk on water. That's just an observation on my part, but it could save you some unnecessary humiliation.

He expressed his next concern as I was leaving the exam room. He walked up to me with his bookkeeper in tow. He had the order for my labs on a sheet of paper, and pointed it at me. He said, "We have a problem!" Your insurance won't pay for chemotherapy". I don't want to give the impression that he was loud and menacing when he approached me, but I will say his demeanor screamed dismissal.

I had checked with Blue Cross/Blue Shield shortly after I found out about my cancer, and was assured chemotherapy was a covered service, and I told him so. I was totally confused. Then, I realized what the real problem was. Although chemotherapy was a covered service it had to be administered in an outpatient setting. Must have been that his facility didn't meet that particular criterion. In other words, before I left his office he personally, and literally, checked out my financial situation. As I think about it now; he had more information on my financial situation than he had on my cancer. Now, there's a lesson in priorities!

It was clear to me that money was the deciding factor whether he was going to treat me or not. Oncologists make a veritable ton of money with each chemotherapy treatment they administer. At the time it appeared that, if he wasn't going to get in on the real money, he wasn't about to waste his time with me. Am I right about his priorities? Who really knows but the doctor himself? All I can tell you is this; what I've described to you is the way it happened.

I'd had about all I could take for one day. Even in my desperation I didn't feel I should have to jump through hoops to please this man so he would treat my cancer. According to him I was a "dead man walking" anyway, so why should I continue with him. And so, with that, the conversation was over. I hadn't said much to him. However, today the whole conversation would have gone differently. I know more about cancer now, and I know there are choices out there and other doctors who care. Most importantly, I'm not desperate now, and he would have had a crystal clear understanding of my side of the situation. *Crystal clear!*

I left his office confused and without hope. My visit to him cost $370 for less than 15 minutes of dialog. I concluded that I had dealt with a doctor who had very little concern for the cancer patient, and one who sees dollar signs as his Holy Grail. Even back then I knew I had opened the wrong door. I needed help, of that there is no doubt, but I didn't need him. Definitely not him.

You've heard the phrase "You don't pay a doctor for his bedside manner"? Good thing! A doctor like this one would find himself sweeping the corridors of the bowels of Hell if it was up to me. He was the 'short straw'…plain and simple.

I exercised my first right as a cancer patient. I vowed to look for an oncologist with whom I could find some faith and trust. I still had the cancer. I was still alone. I was still frightened. And, I was getting angry. So, I began a new search. A search I still believe I shouldn't have had to make.

## Next...

The second oncologist that I found didn't want to treat me because I lived too far away. There was a distance of 70 miles between us, and she didn't practice in my area. She suggested that I find a doctor closer to me. At least she was decent, and I wasn't charged an exorbitant fee, as it was merely a phone call. I may not have felt any better, but at least my checking account hadn't suffered.

I got back into the phone book again, but had little luck. Looking in the yellow pages for an oncologist isn't the best way to find one. To me, and at that time, it was like looking down the barrel of a gun, and wondering if it was loaded. It was like throwing a dart hoping to hit a bull's-eye at 500 yards...<u>blindfolded.</u>

All I could think of is that I didn't want my life to end, at least not until I could stand in front of that oncologist and gleam with health. We all know we're going to die someday. I just didn't want it to be 'this' day. Besides, although I was in no pain it was of considerable interest to me. I believed that cancer and pain were inseparable, and although I wasn't feeling pain yet...I was afraid I soon would. What would I do about that? I didn't have a doctor. Admittedly, there were other things to worry or think about, but the fear of pain was right on the top of my list.

# The Accident

I was visiting a relative one evening in mid-January that year. We had dinner together and were discussing the whole cancer issue. It felt good to get out of my house for a while, and to have someone to talk with about my problem. However, it was getting late, and so I left their house around ten that evening and headed for home.

A snowstorm had just gone through, which left the roads rutted and slippery. I wasn't feeling comfortable about the road conditions at all, so I slowed down to a near crawl. I was on a slight decline in the road when all hell broke loose, and my car began to spin out of control. It made a complete spiral, went off the road, and hit a tree. I felt and saw things go by in slow motion, and I heard the glass break as my car came to rest upon the small tree. Seatbelts are wonderful things, as I hadn't become too chummy with the windshield. My fingers and toes were still positioned properly, so I surveyed the rest of my situation while the dust began to settle.

I knew I wasn't injured. However, as I looked out the passenger-side window I felt truly blessed. That one tiny little tree had prevented the car from tumbling down a shallow ravine. I carefully opened the drivers-side door, crawled out, and found a house with lights on. They let me use their phone and allowed me to wait inside until the police arrived.

The police didn't issue me a ticket, thank God, and I was fine aside from fractured nerves. The tow truck picked up my car and towed it away. As I thought about my car being towed away I had to wonder what it took to set off an air bag. Think about it...my car had bounced all over rutted snow and ice ruts, spun around, then slammed into a tree. When things came to a stop, my airbag was still tucked neatly away where it was when it was brand new. I'm not complaining. Who wants to be slapped by an airbag? I just thought it should have gone off.

The car was considered a total loss. My little car that had gotten 40-miles-per-gallon of gas was gone. I could get another car, I wasn't hurt, and I hadn't been on the working end of that ravine. If God was with me in my car that night, and He surely was, then maybe He knows why my air bag didn't go off. I don't.

I called a car salesman that I knew, and told him what had happened. I asked him if he would find as good a car as my insurance money would afford me. It took about a week, but he offered me one that was five years old, in good condition, and the price landed just inside my budget. It was a much larger car than my other one had been, so I felt like I was driving a tank as I drove it home. The tires were good, the engine ran, and the radio worked. All was well...I needed that car.

## Back to the search

I got myself on the Internet and looked up everything I could find on cancer. I was going to fight this if for no other reason than for pure spite. However, I felt totally alone, and I wished that Dale could still be with me. But then, who knows, maybe he was.

There is a lot of information out there in cyber space. And, there are a lot of supplements that tout the ability to kill cancer cells. I had to try something. The only other alternative was to sit down and die. However, I didn't buy supplements from the Internet. I just didn't have enough information and everything seemed pretty confusing.

I wanted to talk about supplements with a real person, so I went to the closest health food store and asked for something that could possibly help me with my cancer. A couple of things were suggested, and so I tried two or three different supplements. But, as it turned out, I didn't have enough information about them to continue taking them. I wanted to do something, but didn't know enough about those types of supplements to feel good about treating myself. All I knew was that as long as I was still breathing and putting one foot in front of the other... I had to try.

I couldn't get it off my mind that things shouldn't be going this way. There must be something that I could do about all of this. I was facing lessons in medical dismissal that no cancer patient should ever have to face. However, there are legions of patients that are facing precisely what I faced then, and I'm willing to bet that they're as stunned and confused as I was.

A friend told me about a process in a clinic 70 to 80 miles south of where I live. The process involved removing about a cup of blood from my veins, running the blood through a machine that was supposed to kill some of the cancer cells, then my blood was given back to me via the IV. The theory behind this treatment is much like vaccinations for small pox... I guess. Dead small pox cells are injected into the body; the body recognizes the cells and learns immunity...I guess. I don't know if I ever really believed it would kill the cancer, although I guess it could work for someone...who knows? Surely, I didn't. At least something was happening. All I wanted was a chance to fight.

It didn't take the house doctor long to tell me it wasn't working. The last two visits proved to be the end for those treatments. Once my blood was taken through the IV, the technician couldn't get it to flow back into my vein because, by that time, my blood had gotten too thick. The doctor came in the treatment room and, with worry in his voice, told me I needed to see an oncologist. I told him that I had tried, but that it hadn't worked. I simply didn't know the best way to find one.

We both knew I needed a CT scan, but you need a doctor to order one. I don't know why he didn't offer to order one, but he didn't. There must be a good reason why he didn't, but I didn't ask. All I could think about at the time was that time was not on my side. It was getting toward the end of January, and I had to do something, and so, an idea was born. I wanted and needed a dad-burn CT scan, and I was going to get one...one-way or the other.

## What is a CAT (CT) Scan?

For those who aren't familiar with what a CAT scan is: A CAT scan is an abbreviated name for Computerized Axial Tomography. It is an x-ray procedure which combines many x-ray images with the aid of a computer to generate cross-sectional views and, if needed, three-dimensional images of the internal organs and structures of the body. A CAT scan is used to define normal and abnormal structures in the body. A large donut-shaped x-ray machine takes x-ray images at many different angles around the body. A computer to produce cross-sectional pictures of the body processes these images. In each of these pictures the body is seen as an x-ray "slice" of the body, which is recorded on a film. This recorded image is called a tomogram. "Computerized Axial Tomography" refers to the recorded tomogram "sections" at different levels of the body.

That's a lot of technical language, which may be slightly confusing. So...

Imagine the body as a loaf of bread and you are looking at one end of the loaf. As you remove each slice of bread, you can see the entire surface of that slice from the crust to the center. The body is seen on CT scan slices in a similar fashion from the skin to the central part of the body being examined. When these levels are further "added" together, a three-dimensional picture of an organ or abnormal body structure can be obtained.

Better?

## My first CT Scan!

After I left the clinic I didn't even go home before I went to my local emergency room. I told them I had cancer, and that I couldn't find an oncologist. I told them about the treatments I had, what had happened with them, and that I needed help. They were afraid that blood clots could have formed, and so they took me in, and gave me my first CT scan.

After the CT scan results were back the doctor came to talk to me. He was kind and warm hearted so he didn't tell me I was going to die, although he must have thought that to be true. I think he just didn't have the heart to tell me. He said what he had to say with as much kindness as he could.

I couldn't have been in a very coherent mood that day, because I don't remember a great deal about what was said. However, I know he didn't go into much detail about the scan in general. He didn't say a great deal about the cancer either, but he did say I was in no danger over the blood clot issue. I know he suggested that I get on some sort of medication for my nerves, but said nothing about seeing an oncologist.

I got the impression that he wasn't used to dealing with cancer patients who were unable to find a doctor. It was as though he was definitely on the spot knowing what the scan said, and knowing I didn't have help. I think he was just sorry we were both in the same room at the same time, because he was concerned about me and couldn't do a single thing to lessen my fears, my cancer, or my doubts. In other words…he was a good and caring doctor who had very little to offer in the way of help. I'll bet he would be surprised to see me now.

After a bit we chatted about other things.

I had given him a run-down of the reasons I hadn't received real treatment up until then, and I told him about the attitude of the oncologist I had seen. He very kindly suggested that some oncologists are quite often rude, but that

I should try to understand that they dealt with death every day. He said some of them loose their compassion because the death issue is difficult for them to take. What?!

Like we don't know how that feels?! You know what I thought? I thought, I'm only going to die once, and I deserved more respect than I was getting!

I have an idea...how about the oncologist accepts the responsibility for his or her own feelings. Shouldn't we be able to depend on our doctors for the rudiments of help, and that he 'first causes no harm'? I believe that is the part of the Hippocratic oath that is the first to be dismissed by some of them. It doesn't take a mental heavy-weight to know that there is real harm caused by those doctors who are rude, have a total lack of compassion, and by those who dismiss a cancer patient without even a hint of hope. What would happen if they treated me? I *could* die? What would happen if they didn't treat me? I *would* die! Is that so difficult to reason out??

Where are my rights in all of this? I guess I don't know where to buy chemotherapy drugs. But, they do. I don't believe that I would know the proper way to administer them if I could buy them. But, they do. I'll bet that BC/BS wouldn't pay for the drugs unless I have a license to buy them. But, I don't have a license to do that. So, even though I hadn't done anything that could be construed as being wrong, I hadn't broken a law; I was sentenced to death. And, I had to pay exorbitant fees to have the sentence delivered. Gee...shouldn't they, at least, do that for free?

How about we just cut to the chase and they allow me the right to fight for my own life. If I die because I've fought and lost, then they can stand over me at my funeral and say, "I told you so!" See, at that point I wouldn't care. But, as long as my body still functions, my brain still has the ability to think and make decisions, and as long as I'm willing to go for life, then it really ought to be my choice. And, by the way...

Am I wrong, or are hospitals 'not' allowed to refuse treatment when a patient needs help but has no insurance or money to pay for his or her medical treatments. If there are laws against that sort of thing, then where is it written that oncologists can turn cancer victims away...you know...the old 'go home and die' thing? How about some thought be given to that scenario as well!

Let's give some serious thought to this...how about I decide whether I want to fight for my life or give up and roll over! What if the doctor traded places with me for a New York minute? You know, just long enough for him to feel the same kind of fear and dismissal his cancer patients feel.

And that's just about as much empathy for oncologists that I had right about then. As kind as the ER physician was, he didn't have the consideration to help me dig for help either. Certainly, he had a string or two that he could have tugged on to get me started in the right direction toward some sort of assistance, but all he really wanted to see was my back going out the door. Why didn't he help? Who knows? What I did end up with was just enough anger that became the catalyst that some of us need to get something constructive under motion. I was feeling the futility of the whole situation and needed a reason to end my self-indulgence. Dang... I was really angry! Can you tell?

## Where do I go from here?

I made a call to The Cancer Treatment Centers of America. The lady I spoke with was very kind, sounded hopeful, and seemed interested. "Whoopee!" I thought. The conversation was going fairly well until she learned that, although I had BC/BS coverage, I had no insurance coverage for office calls and prescriptions, and no husband to foot the bill. She simply said she couldn't help me either. I guess that surprised me a little, but not much. *To heck with her...*

I was back to the waiting game, and other things. As far as I knew there was no hope and I was going to die... according to my oncologist (Mr. Wonderful) anyway. I hadn't provided a good home for my dog, so I set about doing that, but came up empty. He's a chocolate lab that is convinced he's a human. Or, maybe he thinks we're all dogs. Either way, he had it all figured out.

I realized the best solution would be to have him put to sleep because I couldn't find a loving home for him. He was getting old, and I wasn't about to just dump him where he may not be treated well. But, in the end, I couldn't do it. I began to think he was watching me, with suspicion, out of the corner of his eye. You can't fool dogs and children. They're way too smart for us. I guess I felt that he was in the same situation that I was in only he didn't have cancer. How could he live without love any better than a human could? I didn't know what to do about him.

I couldn't think of anything else to do for myself either. I thought there should be some sort of treatment out there that would help with the cancer, but I had no clue where to find it. I guess I felt that I had tried everything I could think of, and I thought that it was beginning to appear that there really was no hope. I couldn't truly give up though, although I didn't know where to turn. Then, I remembered a friend.

## The third oncologist

I contacted a friend, Joan, who works in a medical office. I asked her if she knew of an oncologist with whom she would deal if she found herself in my situation. I was given a name with the assurance that he was very good. She offered to contact my family doctor, the surgeon who did the biopsy, and the oncologist for any medical records that were available and pertinent. She would have them sent to this new oncologist so the information would be there for the consultation. That would likely eliminate lost time and save another costly office visit. I was elated!

I had only a week or so to wait to see the new oncologist, and looked forward to the possibility of getting some sort of treatments begun. However, as I sat in this new doctor's office I was told he had no information on me at all. It became obvious the requests Joan had made were lying on desks somewhere collecting dust. Fancy that... The only thing we had was the written copy of the emergency room's CT scan that I had in my purse, and so he read it.

When he finished reading the scan, he gave me a pretty thorough examination; you know...the kind where it was obvious he was serious about it. After I was dressed he came back in the examination room. With concern in his voice he said the magic words...words that I hung on for dear life. He said, "Elaine, I may not be able to cure you, but I'm going to do my very best to get you back to normal." See? Compassion! How hard was that!

I couldn't say a word. Finally, I found a doctor who seemed to care. I broke down and cried. He thought my tears were brought on from fear. Fear had nothing to do with my tears at that point. I was finally getting some help from a doctor who cared, and it was the mother of all relief.

He told me about the cancer in my colon, and talked a bit more about the immediate danger with respect to the cancer's location. It needed to be addressed as quickly as possible, he said. I didn't get the impression that he thought treating my cancer was beyond his reach of expertise, or that he thought treating it would be a waste of time. And, by the way, he didn't seem overly concerned about my financial situation, nor did he ask to be put in my will. I needed a couple of tests ran that would help provide the information he needed to treat my cancer properly. Before I left his office he said he would order a bone scan and a PET scan. Again...was that so difficult?

## What is a PET scan?

The acronym 'PET' stands for Positron Emission Tomography and is an examination that involves the acquisition of physiologic images based on the detection of radiation from the emission of positrons. Positrons are tiny particles emitted from a radioactive substance administered to the patient. The subsequent images of the human body developed with this technique are used to evaluate the cancer. When the PET scan finds cancer it measures the cancer in terms of density. That was a mouth full!

Within two week's time both the bone and PET scans were done. In addition, my emotions settled done some, and life seemed a little brighter. Joan had found a living, breathing doctor for me who seemed to care and was willing to help.

While I waited for my appointed time to see the oncologist once more, I relaxed some. Sure, I knew the cancer was still there, that it appeared to be fairly dangerous, and that the road ahead was going to be a rough one. But, somehow I just knew that, since I had a doctor who was 'in this thing with me' I had a good chance to live. I could fight. I knew I could do that. And, now I had a way to fight. Hope reigns eternal, doesn't it?

When I returned to him for the results of the scans I was told I had late-stage, stage-4, aggressive, cancer of the colon. I thought I should have had a calculator to keep track of all the places where cancer had taken up residence in my body, because there was a bunch of it. It had metastasized to the liver, kidney, lymph nodes, adrenal gland, blood, and the soft tissue. There was a tumor by my aorta, and the bone scan showed a cancerous spot in the bone of my left leg. If I had

had as much money as cancer I could have retired comfortably. Including the tumor in my leg, the count was up to nine. I don't know if I felt 'doomed' or not. I don't know if I felt much of anything at that moment.

I don't know how well I emotionally digested the results of the PET scan. It's odd, I guess, that I didn't fall apart. But, I didn't. Something seemed to take over in my soul. It was as though the doctor had been talking about, and to, someone else. I didn't feel much of anything, although I was shaking like a leaf. However, I finally had some answers that I felt I needed, but obviously not the answers I wanted.

At least, I thought, this doctor was going to give my cancer his best shot. I felt I could trust him, and he was kind. I wasn't happy about what he had to say, but he gave me the hope I had been looking for. I began to feel a spark of courage again. I might even have had a glint of hope in the system that I had learned to refer to as the "Cancer Mill". Maybe it *could* work after all.

I thought about colon cancer and the fact that it had spread to eight other areas of my body. And, it appeared to me that I had bone cancer as well. I had two types of cancer at one time? This cancer issue just seemed to be getting worse and worse. I asked the doctor how that could happen, and he explained why that wasn't the case.

He said when cancer spreads to another parts of the body the new tumor has the same kind of abnormal cells and the same name as the primary tumor. For example, if colon cancer spreads to the bone, the cancer cells in the bone are colon cancer cells. The disease is metastatic colon cancer (it is not bone cancer).

At the time I didn't seem to grasp what difference that could make, or why that should be good news for me. But, it does make a difference, and it's huge. Because there was only one type of cancer the drug regime would be the same for each cancer site. That is why it is so very important that the site where the cancer originated be determined. And, it is of paramount importance that the original diagnosis be correct. I wondered if that tidbit of information would be of interest to my first oncologist. However, first he would have to view that as a real issue. The point here is that there are as many drugs for cancer as there are types of cancer, and the drug has to match the cancer type in order for it to work.

Within the next two weeks he wanted me to have a colonoscopy and to see a surgeon. He set up the appointment for the surgeon, and I left for home with some hope. I wasn't sure what sort of treatments would be ordered, or how I would be effected by them. I was sure, though, that I was finally on my way to the fight.

However, two weeks came and went with no appointment for a colonoscopy. I thought it was possible the oncologist had misspoken himself, or that I hadn't heard him correctly. Maybe I would have the colonoscopy after the first visit with the surgeon. I kept my appointment, and wondered what might happen next. I should have known, but am glad I didn't. Knowing what's in the immediate future isn't always a good thing.

## The Surgeon

The surgeon's nurse showed me to the examination room, told me the doctor would be right with me, and then left. I wasn't told to get into a hospital gown in preparation for an examination. Strange, I thought. It must be because the oncologist had given the surgeon information that would eliminate a physical examination during this visit, although that seemed unlikely. Or, it may have been that the examination would come after the colonoscopy was done. Still, it was just odd. So, there I sat in the examination room when the doctor breezed in. He sat down and it began.

The very first words out of his mouth were, "I <u>*won't*</u> treat you." Not, "hello". Not, "How the heck are you?" Nothing. Just, "I won't treat you."

You know how a million thoughts pass through your brain in a matter of seconds? Some are rational, and some are not. Mine were mixed, irrational, and confused. To me, at that very moment in time, "I won't treat you" was a complete dismissal of my existence. At that very moment, my life, my body, how I felt, and my very subsistence had become totally useless because I was sick. Whatever I am, had been, or ever could be meant nothing. It took only one other human being to strip me of my very worth. One other human being made it his right to sentence me to death, and it took only four words to do it. He assumed all the rights where my health was concerned. As far as he was concerned, I had no rights. Hope evaporated. I had just wanted someone to try. How hard could that have been?

I looked at him and asked, "Why?" I was dumbfounded, and I was crushed.

He said he *wouldn't* treat me because there *might* be more cancer in my liver than showed in the PET scan. What did he mean...might? How could he say *might* when my very life depended on him? And, by the way...what happened to the damned colonoscopy!?

Dale's brother, Reg, was with me for that appointment, (where would I have been without his support?) He asked the surgeon why the cancer in the liver couldn't be surgically removed, as he had heard the liver was the one organ that could regenerate itself. If Reg knew that...and the doctor didn't...then what was I doing there?

The doctor's answer was that 'he' *wouldn't* do it. If *might* wasn't conclusive enough for us than *won't* would have to do, as there were no other explanations offered. He implied the notion that it was either 'him' or nothing! Yea...Right!

He said that, if I liked, he would do the surgery on my colon to remove that cancerous tumor. He would not, however, treat the rest of the cancer. Does that make sense to you? Of course it doesn't! Weeks later it would become very clear why that surgery could have meant death for me had I grabbed that particular straw. The idiot!

Again, how about a little research, or maybe some testing would be nice. What gave him the right to sentence me to death without a little legwork on his part? Just who did he think he was!? Self-pity flew past him and out the window. I was beginning to get very angry.

Then, out of the blue, he told me I could call the Mayo Clinic, if I wanted, and ask them to treat me. "However", he said, "They won't treat you." He said he knew this because he had trained out there and knew how they worked.

Where had that come from? Mayo Clinic hadn't even crossed my mind until he brought it up. I wanted to slap him up along side his arrogant head, but I just sat there pretty much crushed. I thought, how could that stupid man say those things to me when he hadn't done the colonoscopy or examined me in any way? I was too confused to think it out clearly. I was too hurt to reply. I wanted to cry and I couldn't. I had to think…

Where had he earned the right to use that arrogant demeanor with anyone, *especially* with a cancer patient? Furthermore, it was apparent he had done little or no research into the cancer that was in <u>my</u> body! Also, it was crystal clear that he had no concern, whatsoever, as to what I might be feeling. The last I knew you could find my heart, soul, and the nasty cancer in the same general area. However, he didn't recognize that fact. It didn't matter, though, because he wasn't willing to treat any part of me.

When the good doctor stopped long enough to take a breath, I asked him how much time I had. He said he didn't know, but that I needed to go home and get my affairs in order.

That's it? No examination, no explanation, no colonoscopy, nothing but 'go home and die'? I mentally told him I would go home and die just as soon as he did! I should have said it out loud. I had, after all, nothing else to loose. But, by that time, I wasn't thinking about anger; I was thinking about dying.

It was apparent to me that it wasn't his position to treat the cancer anyway. It was his job to do the colonoscopy, give the oncologist his findings, and then, do what he was trained to do. You know...surgery? As far as I could tell, he was speaking for the oncologist and a major medical institution with nothing to back up his comments but his inflated ego.

I was shaking so badly this time that my brother-in-law had to make out the check for the office fees. This doctor charged me $161 for his office call. At least the office visits were going down in price. More importantly, it became apparent to me that the oncologist who sent me to the surgeon had taken his word. I never heard from either of them again.

However, in reality, if this doctor had been kind and compassionate with me I could have been in more trouble than I already was. His compassion, or lack of it, wouldn't have changed his outlook on my disease. If he didn't believe I had a snowball's chance in 'you know where' to live through the cancer, then his treatments would likely have reflected that. If I'm right about that, and I believe I am, then I would have died anyway. Where my life is concerned, I needed a lot more support from the doctor than he would ever have to offer. God would lead me where I needed to be, and it didn't appear that this doctor was my optimal destination. I just didn't know that at the time. At the time, I wasn't leaning on God either. That would come a little later, and not a moment too soon.

# Me Time

I went on a pity party whose depths surprised even me. How did I get here? Where could I go? Why isn't "I care" part of their Hippocratic oath? Okay, I've turned sixty, and maybe I'm passed the age of being useful, but didn't my life count for something? Maybe my insurance isn't the best; but I could, I would, and I had paid their hefty fees. Was it that I had a type of cancer that he didn't know how to treat? Was that the cause of the surgeon's abrupt rudeness? And, if he couldn't treat my cancer then why didn't he send me to someone who could? What… did I threaten his fragile ego? Why wasn't *I* given the choice to fight for *my* own life? He wasn't giving <u>his</u> life away; he was giving <u>my</u> life away!

I was hanging on a sapling over the edge of a very large cliff, and the medical community wasn't listening to my cry for help. How many other patients were facing this? I would like to think I was the only one, but I knew I couldn't be. So, there I was …stunned and numbed all over again. Why in the world couldn't I find a little help?

## The End of the Road

After this particular blow I went home to think all of this over. I knew I couldn't fight this thing anymore. I just didn't see how or why I should. I was, by this time, more afraid of life than death. Morbid? Sure, but life gets like that sometimes.

I was painfully aware of how dangerous the cancer was, and that there was no more help now than when it was first diagnosed months ago. I had wasted too much time and paid too much money to a world of people who couldn't have cared less. I was face down, and all rational thought was floating somewhere out of reach. I thought I had calmed down now, but my hands still shook. I couldn't remember to eat, sleeping wasn't easy, and I was drenched in a complete sadness. When I wasn't feeling sorry for myself... I was livid!

I couldn't talk about this to anyone because I didn't know what to say. What do you say to someone when they ask how you're doing? I felt like asking how much time they had, or if they really wanted to know. I wanted to be John Wayne. I wanted to be brave, but I wasn't. I wanted an angel to appear and say things would be fine. But, it wasn't time for an angel yet. I wanted to cry, but couldn't, and I wanted to feel safe. I went through my days smiling while assuring everyone I was just fine because I wanted to be fine. But, it was a big fat lie. *I wasn't fine!*

And then...I gave up.

I called my family and told them what was going on, got my suit cleaned, visited the funeral home and planned my funeral, made out a will, then sat down and began the wait.

## Getting used to death

By now my view of life had made a drastic change. Death wasn't the monster anymore. It actually seemed friendlier than life. Rational thought was not even a concern, and I had no more fight left in me. I couldn't find a doctor who cared if I lived or died, and I'm ashamed to say, I wasn't even sure it mattered. I believe in heaven, and was looking forward to being there. However, I had to die first. By now, the only thing that really frightened me was going through the dying process, and going through it alone. But I was given no other choice, and no one seemed to be capable of, or willing to help me.

The important question now was...how does a person die of cancer? You know...what really happens? How much pain is involved, how long will it take, and when will it happen? Will I know when I'm about to take my last breath? Would I be terribly afraid when the last moment of life arrived, or would I just peacefully slip away? I just didn't know, and I needed to know. *I was scared.*

What really happens can influence some pretty gruesome mental images. But, it became a real curiosity. One I began to dwell on. I'd like to mention here that I was not suicidal, just thinking... I think. Well...I didn't have to be suicidal just then anyway.

I lived alone then, which caused some screwed up thoughts like, "When I died how long will it take for someone to find me?" But then, how much would that have mattered? It wasn't like I was going to face a huge mood swing because I had lost my body. I realized that that particular difficulty was a crisis that someone else would be dealing with. I almost felt sorry for them, and I would have if I hadn't been feeling so sorry for myself.

As it turned out I wasn't the only one whose thoughts were running wild. I had to have house keys made for three of my best friends. They would pop in so often I thought a revolving door should be installed. One of them, Bryan, rented warehousing space from me. He would knock on the door every single day after his route was finished. He had a 'big rig' food route, and before he went home to his wife, a hot meal, and some solitude, he would pop in just to make sure I was okay. And, you know what? That helped.

Linda was another friend who I depended upon to the extreme. I knew I couldn't handle giving Dale's clothes away. It wasn't just that I didn't want to... I couldn't. I knew it had to be done, and I simply didn't have the emotional strength to face that. So, she came over one day while I was gone somewhere and took care of his things for me. She saw to it that people who were in need of clothing were the ones that were helped with his things.

Chuck and Joan worried that I wasn't eating properly, so I would find myself with trays of food every now and then.

And then, there is Danita. She's a lovely, perky young lady who has a perpetual smile on her face. The children she works with have as much love and respect for her as she has for them. As happy-go-lucky as she seems, she is a deep thinker and she feels just as deeply. She came to my house one day totting two cement feet under her arm. They were, she said, to be put where I could see them every day to remind me that all I had to do was put one foot in front of the other. She said she *knew* I could make it.

With all my heart and all my soul...I ask God in heaven to bless all of their souls. At that time my friends were the glue that held me together.

Are you a friend of a cancer patient? Are you wondering how to approach them now that they are sick? I know... I've felt the same way. What if you say the wrong thing? How can you tell them how you feel without making them feel sad? What can you really say, and how do you say it?

Want some advice? Tell them how sorry you are that they have cancer. Give them a hug if you want to; a hug will be welcomed. After that...don't treat them like they are sick. Their love doesn't have cancer. Neither does their sense of humor, nor their need for your friendship. Being there for them in love and spirit is what they're looking for, that's all they really want. If they don't loose your companionship it will help them with their will. Just love them like you always have. That will be enough.

I would like to make a comment for church members. My pastor sent me a book once, and called me on the phone a couple of times. But, other than that, no one from my church visited or called me. Instead, it was a sweet lady, Lou Ann, from another church who came to see me, called on the phone, and sent me e-mails. I thought about that during those times, and I was rather hurt by their absences. I don't think their absences meant that they didn't care about what I was going through. What I do think is that they may have considered it the pastor's duty to do that sort of thing. Must be that the pastor thought it was the congregation's duty to cover that area. The fact is *no one* did. It's a lesson in how to lose a member of the congregation in a hurry. It's the reality of dismissal that bothered me, but I had more pressing matters on my mind to worry much about it.

## Dealing with Death

I guess that everyone has thought about death, for one reason or another, during his or her life. I know I have. But this time I had to face it. It was coming at me with a force of a freight train. There is nothing pleasant about it, and its presents cause a lot of questions and feelings to manifest themselves. I couldn't stop the thoughts no matter how hard I tried. I had to admit that death really did frighten me even though life had begun to frighten me more. I knew that I needed to look for some answers. I had to become part of it in order to understand it.

I wasn't alone in my sorrow. My son was right there with me, and had his church in Georgia praying for me every day, as did my mother's church in North Carolina, and the church I attended at the time had me on their prayer list as well. Friends and acquaintances had Christians from all over the country praying for me too. However, that was the only reality I had to fill the eternity between one moment and the next.

I wanted to be solid in my faith in prayer, but it was apparent that I needed something more. I needed to understand what was about to happen. Faith and understanding would, somehow, see me through if I could just understand death. And, maybe if I could understand death, my faith would become stronger.

## Looking for Answers

I thought if I could share my thoughts with someone maybe I could look at the inevitable a little more objectively. So, I began to look to friends for support and understanding.

People, in general, can talk about life and living all day long. When the subject of death is broached, however, the mood changes dramatically. I don't blame anyone from shying away from the subject, because our own death is a scary business. Talking to me about death was compounded because it wasn't a supposition. Real and imminent death was right on the other side of our conversation, which made it tangible for both of us; not just me. My friends wanted so much to help, so they listened, and they tried to comfort.

In our conversations one of two distinct scenarios came to bear. Either I was giving up, which I couldn't do and still remain in the fight for my life. Or, I was dwelling on a possibility that wasn't going to happen anyway. Either way it was my responsibility to take my mind off of death and think ahead to living. Which, of course I couldn't do. And, that's where the difficulty really lies. Somehow a terminal cancer patient has to keep fighting for life while the doctors, whose prognosis carries a veritable ton of weight, are telling them that there is no hope. How could I get around that? It was a conundrum at best.

Then, the other reality is that our fears are our own. There are people who have just plain gotten tired of life, and who would be very happy to see it come to an end. I couldn't agree, nor understand, that point of view. I didn't see it that way at all. And, the way I saw it was pretty much the way most others look at death as well. It became apparent that the over-all view was that life is difficult enough without making it worse by talking about death.

In the end, talking about death with others didn't seem to solve much of anything. No one really knows much about it, nor what to say on the subject. None of us had experienced it yet, and no one was in any particular hurry to experience it. Nope...death is not a subject that people are pleased to discuss. All but a very few view their own death as anything but cheerful; I was no exception. So, all we can really do is just support the one who is facing death with as much love and compassion as we know how to give. And, that is what I got in those conversations: Love and compassion.

A new way to search took me to the library. I borrowed books on all of the subjects I thought would help me accept dying, and then death. I read anything I could find on death, heaven, dying, being good, being bad, mentally searching my past to list all the people I would have to ask for forgiveness (that burned a fair amount of time), and I read the Bible about things that didn't seem to relate. Which says a lot about where my priorities were up until then.

I found quite a lot of information on NDE's (Near Death Experience). I had read some on this subject in the mid-eighties, so I knew a little about it. Some people who have gone through a short scuffle with the dying process, and were revived, have been given a glimpse of the other side of life via an NDE. Talk about a rainbow at the other end! Now, there's hope you can hang your hat on.

My own father had had an NDE when he was six years old. He told me about it just weeks before he died of heart failure in 1987. He thought it was just a dream, but a dream he had never forgotten. He had never mentioned it to anyone before, he said, because people would have thought he had lost his mind, or worse yet, that he was lying. The thought of my dad lying was so ridiculous it was almost funny.

I thought of the old western movies I'd seen as a little girl. Do you remember the ones where the Indians would lay a hot knife on someone's tongue as a test of their honesty? Thing was, if your mouth was dry your tongue would burn and brand you as a liar. If not, the hot knife would do no harm, which proved you were telling the truth. I certainly hoped that particular process was nothing more than Hollywood's imagination. God forbid that someone had actually tried it. Moreover, I felt truly blessed that Dad and Mom hadn't used those tactics, as; during my teenage years my tongue would have taken a real beating. A point that I would rather forget...but haven't so far.

The rational here is that honesty was very important to my Dad. I didn't want his dream to be a wonder to him anymore. So, I told him I thought it was a real event (because I did), and referred him to Dr. Moody's book, *Life After Life*. Dad was a cool guy. Whether he read the book or not didn't matter, he knew I believed in him and his *dream*. Shortly after our discussion he died. He was just such a good dad. I'm selfish enough to wish he were still alive. He is truly missed by those of us who loved him.

After much reading, and renewed faith in life after death, I was able to come up with my own little theory on the whole matter, and my theory is this: (It's a little complicated, so I'll try to write slowly ☺).

Life isn't supposed to be easy, and it isn't. Once you've accepted that fact, once your expectations aren't so lofty then life, and ultimately death, seems easier to get through. As you know, no theory is 100% accurate. So, I thought that after you've 'fought the good fight' doesn't it seem fair that there should be a trade-off? Difficult life...easy death? When my time comes I would like to be as healthy as a horse one day, go to bed happy, fall into a peaceful sleep, and then just not wake up. That worked for me. So, I had to beat cancer to be healthy, because I had to be healthy in order to die the way I had it planned. Okay...I know what you're thinking, and I won't argue...because you're probably right. Oh, to be rational again...

In the end understanding the whole situation was some-what helpful, I guess. But, it wasn't the all-in-all answer I'd hoped for. So, I decided to do what I should have done way back in November. I handed my whole life, with all its fears, desperation, and irrational thoughts over to God. I've never taken it back. Please note here that, knowing what I've learned by doing this, I deeply regret that it took me so long to put my life in God's hands. I could write volumes on that subject alone, but I won't. Except to say this... I read some-where that just going to church doesn't make me a Christian any more that standing in my garage makes me a car. That's a cute way of stating a profound truth. Merely handing my life over to God doesn't mean He can take it over unless I let Him do that on a daily basis. Then, I have to listen to Him. Having been born a female, listening can be somewhat diffi-cult at times. If you're a guy, you'll appreciate that.

A week or so passed and I began to get some solace back, although, at the time I didn't have a clue where it was coming from. It was only later when I realized that my prayers for courage, strength, and faith were answered the moment I asked God for them. Moreover, God took the weight of my life from me. I found it profound when I realized that God's way, His promise of friendship and strength, and the comfort I received because of it was all I really needed. I didn't ask Him to heal my cancer, as I knew He would if it was His will, and whatever He decided for me was okay. *It really was.*

I know that many of you are shaking your head, as you've known that having faith in God is where real peace and love is found. I could call myself a late bloomer. But the fact is, if I hadn't had these trials to deal with, I doubt that I would have ever really 'gotten it'. God did not give me this cancer to teach me a lesson. God didn't give me this cancer at all. However, I believe He has used the opportunity to prove His love for me.

I had talked about death, researched it, tried to envision what it might be like, and then prayed about it. I had done all I knew how to do. It was settled as well as it could be. Finally, I was...okay.

# Help... A Reason to Fight

It was during that time, near the end February, when my brother came to see me (Thank you Duane). He suggested I contact Karmanos Cancer Treatment Center in Detroit. He and my sister-in-law, Karla, had done some research and found them to be one of the best cancer treatment centers in this part of the country, (although I had never heard of that particular cancer center, their expertise and caring support would become blazingly clear to me a little later). It took me less than a split second to think of that as a good idea. So I called for, and was given an appointment. It was a 220-mile trip one way to the center, but it was hope. I hoped that the trip to Karmanos would bring better results than I had seen up until then.

It's interesting to note here that hope can be found even when you think you've used up the very last drop of it. When you become too desperate or emotionally wrung out to even look for it. Hope is still there busily building itself up a reserve just waiting to be tapped once more. Duane and Karla weren't thinking so much in terms of hope as they were my survival. But, it's all mixed up together. I'd come to realize that you really couldn't have one without the other. I had begun.

## Gentlemen: Start Your Engines!

I had a lot to do to get ready for my appointment in Detroit, and had very little time to get things done.

Remember I told you that Dale and I had a business? Well, that meant that I would have to leave everything at home and unprotected to stay with my brother and sister-in-law for quite a while. I would be absent for the frozen water pipes in the winter. Oh darn, huh? Everyone would know I wasn't home, and there were thousands of dollars worth of equipment that I couldn't keep an eye on. Not to mention all the 'stuff' in our home. In the midst of all of this I had to close the business until I was back on my feet, and I still had to find a good temporary home for my dog Bubba.

Chuck Connell, Joan's husband, has been a good friend to both Dale and I for years. He established Children's Charters some years ago. Children's Charters is his way of helping kids who want to hunt and fish, but have no one to go with or to teach them how. He has very little money, but he uses what he can to support his effort. I wonder if he realizes just how much of a spiritual gift he is to those children. The children's look of triumph as they drag in a four-inch lunker surely wasn't lost on me, and I doubt that it was lost to him either.

Chuck was broken up over Dale's death, and just as concerned about my cancer. When he found I had finally found some hope he offered to take care of things until I got back home. I asked him if he would take care of the other 'things', such as the funeral and the legalities of my will if I didn't make it back home. He said he would do anything he could. It was no easy task for him, but he dealt with it very well. I felt total relief and blessed, and was truly thankful.

Next, I had to get the information that Karmanos wanted. That included all the available records, scans, biopsy reports and slides, opinions, and whatever else I could get me hands on and bring it all to the first appointment. I began to accumulate as much as I could as fast as I could.

One of the receptionists at one of the doctor's offices asked where I wanted the records sent. I gave her the name of my doctor and Karmanos' address.

"Oh", she said. "I have that address."

It took me a second to realize she knew all about the treatment center, who the doctors were, and where they were. If she knew, I thought, then it was a pretty good bet that the doctor knew as well. Okay, why hadn't they referred me? Why wasn't I given that choice! Surprise and anger got all mixed together and surfaced. It was purely a knee-jerk reaction.

I said, "Then the doctor knows about Karmanos?"

"Oh, sure, we send patients down there all the time", she said

Well…now I'm livid all over again, but considered with whom I was speaking. She had nothing to do with the decisions that had been made, so I gritted my teeth and said nothing. However, any remnant of faith I could have had in this particular doctor evaporated. I felt blessed that he wasn't going to be involved in any treatment I may eventually receive.

## Don't be afraid

I had an unusual experience as I was on my way home that day. I wasn't thinking about much of anything, you know how it is when your mind goes into overload… when it has had enough. I didn't *want* to think. I was neither in a good or a bad mood. I was just driving along looking at the scenery, watching my driving, and actually enjoying the quiet.

The only way I know how to describe what happened is that I had and 'audible thought'. It was not just a passing thought, not something that my mind conjured up, nor was it something I could actually hear. All I remember 'sensing' was; "Don't be afraid." That's all there was..."Don't be afraid". A peace that is difficult to convey washed over me after that. I knew that either I would die in a peaceful way, or the cancer was going to be cured. Either way, I knew I had nothing to fear. One way or the other I was going to be okay.

I was emotionally and physically exhausted when I got home from the 'gathering' of records. I flopped down on the couch and went to sleep within seconds, and I dreamed of my late husband. It was that sort of dream that put you *there*. It was as real to me as reality itself.

In my dream I saw him standing near by. I went to him and twisted his shirt in my fists to get him closer because I was so happy to see him. He just looked at me with a smile and held me in his arms. That was it. Then, I woke up.

In my dream he glowed. I mean there was a sort of aura around him, and I thought how healthy he looked. He looked younger than when he died, but it was Dale nonetheless. The dream will always be a total comfort to me. It was the sort of *real* that made me realize that Dale was okay. He was happy, and he was okay. I wasn't sad for him anymore, I was actually very happy for him. I still missed him though.

## The Consultation in Detroit

I took the first of many trips to my brother and sister-in-laws home in Monroe, which is just south of Detroit. I would stay with them for a few weeks if this oncologist worked out. If he did, Duane promised to take me to office visits, hospitals, treatment centers, and wherever else I was sent. He assured me that he would take care of me and do what ever was necessary to get me back to health. Together, Karla and Duane would do the "God thing" and promised to support me in every way they could.

I had as much information with me as I could lay my hands on when Duane took me for my first consultation with the oncologist at Karmanos. This doctor was kind, informative, and appeared to be willing to help. Whether he could actually help or not was still up in the air. He wanted his own tests ran. If, and how, he could help would be determined by those tests. At least, he was willing to give me the chance to fight for my life. As you might guess, it was a starting point of *epic* importance to me.

Finally! This is just what I had been looking for. He didn't waste time getting a healthcare regime in motion either. He set up appointments for another CT scan and a PET scan at a major hospital. He ordered a colonoscopy, and set up an appointment with a colorectal specialist in Southfield. Just think of all those tests, an appointment for a colonoscopy, and a consultation with a surgeon who specialized in colorectal issues. And, all of this would be seen to in one week's time. Un-swearword believable!

The beginning had begun.

During all of the testing, every nurse and technician I dealt was so very kind and patient, and they answered any question that they were able to answer. I thought, "So this is where the good and caring medical people were hidden!" Who knew! They were within 220 miles of home, but well within my reach. I settled down some, and my will-to-live began to resurrect. Hope promised to spring to life, and my thoughts seemed willing to take a gamble on trust. This new promise got my undivided attention.

Duane was with me through all the scans, blood labs, and all the question and answer sessions. After all the necessary tests were taken we were ready for my next visit with the oncologist. The results of the tests, and the second visit with the doctor was to take place on the following Monday.

However, the doctor who was supposed to read the tests was at an important seminar, which was being held out of state. The scheduler had been unaware of his absences when she set up my appointment. He was the only doctor on my oncologist's list that was allowed to determine the test's outcome, so I had to wait another week for the next appointment date to arrive before I found out what the results were. That, my friends, was a very...very long week.

Before we left for my next appointment, I had a heart-to-heart with Duane. I told him that I finally had the chance to fight for my life, and I finally had a doctor who seemed to care enough to at least try, and that I was totally grateful for all of that. But, most importantly, I had a living breathing person who loved me and was willing to stand with me through it all. I thanked him for being that person. However, I told him that at that moment I felt more frightened of the effects I would suffer from the chemotherapy treatments than of the cancer itself. He turned around and looked at me, and he said, "If other people can do it, you can". He gave me an understanding smile, and I knew I had to swallow the fear. And, that was that.

It's an odd thing about fear. When I had to face fear alone it took over my whole life. It was the source of power that riveted me in hopelessness. Any tomorrow I might have had was dark and bleak. But, when I could share my fear with Duane, it became manageable. Somehow, sharing my fear with my brother made me feel less venerable and less alone. It allowed me to take a step out of that empty space that I had learned to live in.

And now, the time had finally arrived when I would learn which road my future would take. I would either go back home to wait out the days I had left, or I was on my way to the battle that could save my life. I was emotionally sweating in anticipation.

When the doctor met us in the examination room he went over the reality of the tests that had been taken. I was told that I had *less than two months to live without chemotherapy*. Also, he told me that the only reason he would treat me was that I had a strong body. He warned that if I decided to go on, I should understand that chemotherapy is successful only 50% of the time. Then, he added; if my cancer *could* be put into remission, I would only get it back. In the end I would die of this cancer. Time was all he could offer. That may sound pretty bleak, but I had to think about what he was offering. He told me straight out what was ahead of me. But, he also gave me the *choice* to fight for my life. He offered all of his knowledge and compassion, he promised the same from his associates, and he allowed me to believe that my life still meant something. This was where hope took the lead. This is when I was allowed a part in my recovery. And, this is when compassion reigns. And that came straight from the heart.

After giving me all the information that I needed to make an informed decision, what happened next rested solely in my hands. He told me these things in a very professional way, but was kind about it. I don't believe he would have been too surprised if I had chosen to end the battle right then and there, as he knew better than anyone what effects chemotherapy drugs had on a patient's body. If I had decided to put an end to the whole issue I don't imagine he would have suggested against it. I'm guessing he may have offered something to ease the anxiety.

However, anxiety medication wouldn't be necessary. Giving up had never accomplished a single positive outcome on anything for as far back as I could remember. It wasn't even a consideration. Not even close! I was going to fight! All I cared about at the time was that he was willing to fight with intent, and by my side. That's all I asked for. See? That wasn't so difficult, was it?

I asked him what was next. He let us know that anyone who would have any interest in my treatments would be a member of a panel of doctors. That was the reason for the week's delay with my second appointment. Anyone who had any input would include their thoughts to be debated at a round-table setting for all of the doctors to discuss. They would take the value of their combined education, ideas, and thoughts and pool the information into an acceptable treatment. Those treatments would be thought through, and adjusted for my particular cancer and for my particular body. What a concept! No one doctor could put a cog in my life wheel. No one oversized ego would have the right to throw in the first scoop of dirt. No one doctor could take away my hope. *No one could.*

The results of the colonoscopy showed that the opening in my colon was the size of a pencil and was almost blocked off. That, of course, could be deadly (just one of many cheery thoughts). The colorectal surgeon suggested that I have bowel resection surgery as quickly as possible to prevent that from happening. I was in agreement, and was given a run-down of what the surgery would involve. The surgery itself is, these days, fairly commonplace so that wasn't going to be a problem. However, this doctor was part of the mix, and so his suggestion was presented to the panel of doctors at Karmanos for review.

At the next appointment with my oncologist I was given more news and an option to consider concerning the colorectal surgery. There was real danger in waiting out the seven-day recovery time in the hospital after the surgery, and then the four to six weeks of additional recovery time it would take to heal. Chemotherapy is a highly toxic poison, and it would take every ounce of strength my body could muster to stay alive after the treatments began. My body had to be as healthy as possible before chemotherapy could be induced. Taking time out for the surgery would give cancer four to six weeks longer to do more damage. That was more time than my oncologist felt I should risk taking. Actually, it was more time than I had. I had to remember that, at that moment in time, my life expectancy was guessed at approximately two months. It was obvious that aggressive action, along with calculated risk, was in order. The consensus was that it was a reasonable risk to delay the surgery and to get the chemotherapy started as quickly as possible. The cancer was in a rage. I wasn't though. I was beginning to feel alive again.

My brother and I were warned about complications that could present themselves without the surgery. We were given instruction, possible scenarios, and symptoms to watch for. If certain symptoms presented, I could have moments – not hours - to get to the hospital for help. Obviously, none of what was talked about was good news at all, and it appeared to me that the situation was at the point of being desperate. However, I had confidence that, no matter what happened, I would be in capable hands. And, I had the comfort of knowing that I wasn't facing this all by myself.

I would have been happy to have the tumor in my colon surgically removed, just to have that much of the cancer gone. However, the doctor's advice made sense to both of us, so it was agreed that the surgery would take a backseat for the time being. We both had been made aware of the risks, and we were both willing to do whatever was necessary for the best outcome. We were going to see this thing through to the end...together. Treatment for my cancer was just around the corner, and I would like to say here...Yahoo! ☺.

While I was yahooing, Duane was very concerned as it is very difficult to watch someone you love go through what I was going through. But as I said, he was determined to see me through it all. I can't put into words what his support

77

meant to me. It was like he took me from some dark place where there was no escape and put me in a place where it was warm and alive. I wasn't alone anymore. Death wasn't the winner anymore. Fear was in a holding pattern, and there was a tiny glow beginning to warm my belief system. He took me under his arm and wasn't about to let anything happen to me that he could prevent. He was my brother, and I was alive!

## The Battle

I was to understand that a proper course of events needed to be followed in a battle. Otherwise, control over important factions of the fracas could be jeopardized. The next issue caused treatments to be delayed for another few days.

I needed a port implanted. An implantable port is a thin, soft, plastic tube that is put into a vein in your chest or arm and has an opening (port) just under the skin. This allows chemotherapy durgs to be given into a larger vein. The tube is a long, thin, hollow and known as a catheter. The port is a disc about 2.5–4cm in diameter. The catheter is usually inserted (tunnelled) under the skin of your chest. The tip of the catheter lies in a large vein just above your heart and the other end connects with the port which sits under the skin on your upper chest. The port will show as a small bump underneath your skin which can be felt, but not much of it is visible on the outside of your body.

The risk without a port is that the smaller veins of my arm would have to do the work. Please remember that chemo-therapy drugs have a notorious history of collapsing these smaller veins. That would cause complications of monu-mental proportions that I wasn't too crazy about. I have to say, though, that having the chemotherapy drugs adminis-tered so closely to my heart was unnerving. Chemotherapy drugs can, after all, be just as bad or cause death more quickly than the cancer itself. However, at this point in time, I didn't see where I had another choice. It was agreed that the insertion would be done.

This process is done in a hospital's operating room. It is, however, nothing to be too concerned about if it's done properly, as mine was. The process takes about one-half hour unless you request to be put to sleep. That would mean an additional two-hour stay in the hospital to recover from the drugs. The other option was to undergo the port insertion using local anesthetic. I opted for the local anesthetic, as I just wanted to get it over with and get the heck out of the hospital.

Actually, it wasn't too bad (that's my brave side talking). There was no pain involved at all, only some pressure as the work was being done. The pressure may not have caused pain, but it got the attention of my apprehensive side. They tried to make the surgery go less fearfully for me by putting a towel over my eyes in the operating room so I couldn't see what the doctor was doing. Like I would have looked anyway? Not a chance! They couldn't have *made* me look.

A male nurse stood by my side and held my hand through the whole procedure as well. Actually, it was more like he offered his hand so I could crush it for 30 minutes. He was a very brave boy. I'm sure when I felt any pressure, whatsoever, his voice would have reached a higher octave had he uttered a single sound.

I tried to think of something to talk about to keep my mind off of scalpels, very long tubes, and blood...my blood. In other words, I babbled on about nothing. I couldn't see anything but the backside of the towel, so I have no idea how the two men were reacting to my prattle. I didn't hear anything that could be construed as objectionable, so I just keep saying whatever came to mind, and I'm sure it was less then interesting to the two men. Finally, the whole procedure was over and I was allowed to leave.

I was pretty happy with myself after it was over. As you may have guessed, I'm not the bravest person in the world. So, mentally I gave myself an "at-a-girl" while vowing never to do that again. My brother and I left the hospital, and walked out into a beautiful day filled with sunshine. I felt as though the port represented the beginning of my battle; the battle I hadn't thought I was going to have the choice to wage. However, my ego wasn't too happy with the bump the port made in my chest. I'll blame my ego just as if I had no control over it.

## The Work Began...But First; A Moment

Give me just a moment to allow you to know where I was emotionally as the work began. Just a moment to let you know that there was a moment that was plucked from the events that were taking place that lead me to a very critical time. It was a moment where reality slammed up against hope. It was that moment when time stood still until I made a final decision. What could I do about chemotherapy drugs? What would I do? The time had arrived.

All I was offered was time.

Time. Isn't that what we all want? I mean, when it gets right down to the act of dying, when your life is measured in days instead of years, isn't time our first concern? The quality of our lives is surely a major concern. But, I thought; if I could live...if I could have more time, I would worry about quality later. Is that rational? Maybe it is, and maybe it's not. Rationality and reality weren't anymore relative to me than they were when Dale died. If that even makes sense to anyone but me.

I guess the only advice I could take at the time was my own. It was my body, my cancer, my decision, and I was the one who would live with it, or die because of it. It was just an awesomely troubled frozen moment in my life where decisions simply had to be made. They were decisions that gave no room for second chances. They were decisions that literally meant life...or death.

There were a lot of things to think about where these issues were concerned. I would be given a veritable ton of chemotherapy drugs. More drugs, I think, than the average cancer patient gets. Drugs, that I would come to compare to as battery acid. They would be coursing *way* too close to my heart via a port, and the devastation that the drugs would cause could be 'major'. But, I had to think about time, didn't I? I had to live. And, I had no idea there were other options for me. If I had known there were non-toxic therapies that I could take to help me stay healthier during the drug treatments, maybe I wouldn't have been so afraid. But, I just didn't know. All I could consider at the time was killing something that was killing me. And, if killing the monster took chemotherapy drugs, than that was what it took. I wanted to live. I didn't want to give in to cancer. I had to try.

As far as the doctors were concerned, the amount of chemotherapy drugs I would be given wasn't the issue. Nor, was the main concern what the drugs would do to my body; I was going to die anyway. Time was all they could offer me. They were just trying to give me more time. The drugs would work, or they wouldn't.

But, I had to try didn't I? I had a lot of things to consider, and none of the decisions were easy. Not easy at all. So, I took that first step into whatever the future had in store for me. What else could I do? What other options did I have? At that moment...there were no other options.

Now, lets get on with what took place. Let's see if I had made the right decision. Let's rev it up, and let's get going. A little more time was all I needed.

## Here We Go Folks...

During the following office visit the doctor sat down with us to explain what would happen next, and to tell me to be very careful with my leg. He told me that chemotherapy would have no effect whatsoever on the cancer in the bone; it would have to be radiated. In other words, He could do nothing for it. He said that if I broke it, it would never heal. That is NOT a good thing to hear. As you might know by now, I'm not fearless. Somehow, though, I felt the cancer in my leg wasn't going to prove to be a problem. I would address that problem down the road. I could be careful with my leg, and it would be okay for now.

After that, he got into what the chemotherapy treatments would involve. I was to have 51 hours of chemotherapy drugs every other week. 51 hours? I would be given eight hours of a combination of Oxaliplatin, Leucovorin, and Avastin Most of the above would be given in the treatment center, while, one of the chemotherapy drugs was to be given orally. Then, I would be fitted with a 'fanny pack' that I would wear outside the treatment center. It would pump another chemotherapy drug, 5FU, into the port. It would take 43 hours to empty the bag of this chemo drug.

I thought to myself that 51 hours of any sort of drug was an awfully lot to take in. Then, I wondered what 51 hours of chemotherapy drugs could do to my body. Again, unless I wanted to give up and die, that was the only choice I had, and I was *glad* to have that choice. I just hoped that I could live with it. I hoped that I could live through it. I trusted that God wouldn't lead me this far only to have me to loose the battle due to the drugs I had to take. I was beginning to toughen up.

I was taught how to handle removing the fanny pack needle from the port site and how to take care of myself until the next treatment date. I was given all the information

I needed to get things underway. With all of the tests over, most of the concerns addressed, and the information given; it would soon be time to get the actual treatments underway. However, there was one last issue to address.

In general, we were given certain things to be aware of. One of those concerns was a fever that reached 100 degrees. If I got a fever that reached 100 degrees I was to go to a hospital's emergence room immediately. Somehow a fever that low wasn't something I thought an emergency was made of. But then, in the beginning, I couldn't believe I had cancer either. That was a mistake that nearly cost me my life. So, I thought I would err on the side of good sense and pay attention this time.

How could a temperature of 100 be a threat? At the time I didn't fully understand where the chemo drugs drew the line in the sand. I would find out later that they were the General Patton of germ warfare and were calling all the shots. It would take out the enemy, but when the good guys got in the way they were going down just as hard. When that happened my immune system would take a real beating, and pneumonia was very apt to set in. Pneumonia is not the least bit unusual, rather, just a fact of life when cancer patients are in treatment using chemotherapy drugs. Another happy thought...

With the office visit over, the doctor walked Duane and I out to the waiting area where his scheduler was stationed. As he was giving her his orders... it struck me.

I turned to him and said, "How much is the oral chemotherapy drug going to cost?"

He gave me a rather concerned look and said, "Hundreds."

I couldn't say anything. For a second or two I felt my hope begin to drain away again. It wasn't just the oral chemo that was a financial concern; the pills that prevent the horrible nausea were an out-of-pocket cost as well. As memory recalls, those pills are very expensive, and I needed ten of them a month. I didn't have prescription coverage, or that kind of money. It just wasn't there. I just looked at him and said, "Well, I guess that's it then."

Concerned, he asked if I had prescription coverage, and I said, "No, I do not".

Although recent history suggested this situation should have ended any hope of treatments, it didn't. The doctor never skipped a beat. He instructed his scheduler to touch base with my contact person at the treatment center to see what could be done. I...was...floored! I went from elated, to devastated, back to elated again in a matter of seconds. It was one of those moments where your emotions turn you into a human yoyo. Then you're set back into a friendlier, gentler flow. In other words...it was a SHEW moment!

Just think, not only *could* he help me with this disease, he *would* help, and he would actually pull what strings he had to see that it happened. He wasn't going to let money, or the lack of it, be the deciding factor whether I lived or died like the first oncologist implied. My sense of worth began to stir to life again, and I can't tell you how blessed I felt right then and there!

So, how did all this work out? As smooth as butter. The cancer center donated the nausea medication to me, and the order for the oral chemo was changed to the IV type. As long as the chemo flowed through an IV, and was administered on their site, my insurance would cover it. Another boot in cancer's behind. Yes!!

But, I had a problem with the port site. We had waited two weeks for the port site to heal, but it began to look infected. Duane, Karla, and I were concerned that the cancer center wouldn't be able to use the port if the infection proved to be severe. I was very concerned, as I wanted to get the treatments underway. We would find out how that would be handled the next day.

# March 13, 2006 - The Big Day

My first appointment for chemotherapy treatment was an important one for me. I wasn't so fearful; I was just anxious to get things started. After the blood labs were taken I was lead to my chemotherapy booth. There I found a television with the capability of playing movies, a big recliner, books and magazines to read, a blanket and pillow, and an IV pole. All of this was enclosed in curtains for privacy. Cool!

The port site was examined and our fears were realized; it was infected. At first the nurses weren't going to use the port, and talked about using the veins in my arm. However, because I needed the 5FU via the fanny pack, the port was essential to my treatment. Without using the port and the fanny pack, I would be facing a 48-hour stay in the hospital so they could administer the 5-FU. No one, least of all me, thought that was a practical solution. The doctor was called in to take a look. He determined that the port could be used. However, the site was to be monitored closely. After the doctor left the chemo booth the nurses began to get my first treatment underway.

I was given two tablets for nausea and prepped for my first chemotherapy treatment. Each patient has these two nurses in attendance to get the chemo drugs setup and running. I was asked to verify my name and birth date. There were codes and numbers on each chemotherapy dose intended for my treatment that were verified between the two of them, and the process to get the chemo running was double checked as well. Nothing to worry about here, I thought. They left nothing to chance. It was my birthday, by the way. My treatments were finally underway...I thought what a gift that was!

Duane was in my booth with me, and was reading a book. I don't recall whether I was watching television or reading. But, I remember hearing a man coughing and remembered paying little attention to it. All the patients in this room were ill to one degree or the other. I guess my mind considered coughing a natural event considering where we all were. Then, I caught sight of the man. He had a hold on his IV pole and was trying to make it through the opening of his chemo booth. Quickly, there were nurses all around him, and they slid a chair underneath him. Within a minute's time he lost consciousness. His chin dropped to his chest, and the nurses had to hold him in his chair so he didn't fall to the floor. The nurses were in control, but obviously anxious about the man. I heard one call to the other to phone 911. While waiting for an ambulance, the man was in and out of consciousness a couple of times, but, as there were no beds available for him to lie down on, the nurses held him in his chair. When the ambulance took the man away I knew that he was still alive. Another thing I remember about that man is that he was there...alone. He didn't have a friend or a member of his family with him. He was facing this serious emergency... alone. Chemotherapy is not good under any circumstances, it's even worse alone.

When the commotion was over, I asked the nurse what had happened. I was told that this was the man's first chemotherapy treatment, and it was apparent that either he had an allergic reaction to the drugs, or that his body simply couldn't withstand the drugs. I was assured that the man would recover. But, I wondered what he could do about his cancer without chemotherapy drugs to help him. Inasmuch as I was truly concerned about that poor man, I was a little uneasy for myself as well. After all, this was treatment number-one out of twelve treatments for me.

Before my twelve treatments were over, I would see that circumstance repeat itself two more times with two different patients. Without knowing what happened to them, I'm left wondering how they made out.

## The Tough part Begins...

About 48 hours after my first chemotherapy treatment was over my understanding of 100-degree temperature grew by leaps and bounds. I had wanted to go home after the treatment just to see that everything was still okay. So, I took the 220-mile trip to check things out. What a ditz!

You know how illness sort of creeps in, and you don't think much of it until you're ready to lie down in a mass of "woe is me"? When I realized that I truly was getting sick, I also realized that I had a lot of ground to cover to get back where my lifelines were. Why hadn't I used my head! Again! Well, the only thing I could do was pretend I wasn't sick and hit a quick trail for my brother's house. So, that's just what I did.

I was pretty sick when I got back. I found a thermometer and took my temperature. Sure enough, the thermometer read 100 degrees. I found Duane and asked him to take me to the hospital. We were in the car in five minutes time and on our way. I was examined in the emergency room, and then admitted as a patient. I had pneumonia. Drat!!

I had only one treatment behind me with months more ahead, and the chemotherapy drugs were already beginning to wreak havoc on my body. I was unnerved, still determined, but I was a little frightened. As I'm sure you know pneumonia can be very dangerous, even deadly, especially to a cancer patient. *I knew that too...*

And so, I found myself in the hospital. The doctors were aware of the cancer, so they would have to take extraordinary care. Duane was there to see that it happened. Man, it felt good to have him with me! After I was admitted I became very tired, so I just crawled into bed, covered up, closed my eyes and went to sleep. That didn't last long though. Soon a nurse came to my room to take my vitals and get the treatment process begun.

I was urged to try to cough up phlegm in order to iden-tify the strain of pneumonia I had, (sorry, I know that can't conjure up a pleasant mental image). I couldn't do it though. So, the doctors hit the pneumonia with their full arsenal. I don't have a hint of a clue what they had running in my IV, but whatever it was…it was working. On one hand, I began to feel a lot better. On the other hand, all I had to do was roll over and I was upchucking. I looked at it as a fair tradeoff though. Die…or vomit. I have always hated being sick 'that way', but all of a sudden it didn't seem to be much of an issue with me.

You don't spend a lot of time eating when you're in therapy using chemo drugs, nor when you're sick with some-thing else. I was no exception. I was urged to at least try to eat. I thought about trying, but thought, even if I was hungry and tried to eat, it wouldn't have stayed down anyway. I wasn't looking at the long-term benefit that eating would give. I didn't want to eat; I was just tired and I only wanted to sleep, so that's what I did. Cooperation is the name of the game…most of the time.

One of the doctors whose care I was under came to my room one day, and he was upset. He had a similar look on his face as my dad did when he caught me misbehaving. Ahhh, the memories… Anyway, he came to check on me because he felt the other doctors were overdosing me with the antibiotics. It bothered him much more than it bothered me though. I didn't know what overdosing on an antibiotic could cause, but I knew what pneumonia could cause. When I weighed the two options…antibiotics versus pneumonia… I would have chosen the antibiotics.

He had a valid point. Before he took over my treatment I found myself spilling my cookies for no apparent reason. After his visit things got back on a more even keel. I don't pretend to know where the risk was in all of this, and I try not to play doctor, so I don't know if I was ever in any real danger, but I don't know that I wasn't either. I couldn't have been too bad, and certainly better than the pneumonia. He did the right thing. I'm alive to tell about it. Cool!!

Through it all, I felt that I couldn't have been treated with more concern or with better care. Pneumonia had put me in a rather dire situation, but there were a whole troop of doctors who knew exactly what had to be done, and they set about doing it. They didn't ask me how much money I had, where I was from, or if I thought I could handle the treatments. I needed help...and they gave me all the help I needed. I am totally aware of the fact that I literally owe them my life, and I didn't even have a chance to thank them. They were nowhere around the day I was discharged, or I surely would have.

After spending five days in the hospital, I was out in the sunshine again. I was ready for my second chemo treatment in a few days. I might not have felt so hot, but I was alive for the fight that lay ahead. It didn't matter to me where I was; it mattered to me where I was going. This was my rainbow after the rain...there's always a rainbow after the rain. I wasn't just looking at it; I was *in* it.

Just a small note here about cancer, pneumonia, and doctors who either follow the 'book' to closely, or don't follow it at all.

A life-long friend of mine had an uncle who suffered through many treatments of chemotherapy. He worked through all the sickness that goes along with conventional treatments. He had the hope and gritty determination to see his treatments through to the end. After a tough fight, he was declared 'in remission'.

Just as soon as he felt well enough, he and his wife took a little holiday to celebrate. Upon his return home he came down with a case of pneumonia and was admitted to a hospital. Because he couldn't cough up phlegm so the lab could determine which strain of pneumonia he had, they wouldn't medicate him. He lay there… and he died. Their excuse? They wouldn't give him anything for the pneumonia until they could identify the strain. Guess what folks…I couldn't cough up phlegm either. I'm alive today because a group of doctors (along with my brother) weren't willing to let me die.

If the personnel in your hospital won't treat you, then leave and find a hospital that will. Find a doctor or hospital that knows what they're doing and are willing to go the extra mile for you, and don't take no for an answer. It's your right. It's your fight. It's your life!

## Back to my treatments

The second treatment caused acid reflux so intense that I could barely swallow water, as the chemo was burning my esophagus. Budd-dy! You've seen an old used up balloon that is all stuck together. When I tried to swallow it felt like that old balloon that was being ripped apart. That caused some pretty intense pain. Eating anything solid was totally and absolutely out of the question. I know that because I tried. I didn't know swallowing could cause that much pain. I'm here to tell you that it can.

Two chemotherapy treatments down, and a lot more to go… God help us all.

By this time I was driving back and forth from my home to my brother's for my treatments. I had 43 hours before I got 'chemo sick', and I wanted to be home for the event. I was well into my trip home when I called my contact person at Karmanos. I asked her for advice on what to do about this situation. She instructed me to go straight to the hospital's emergency room just a soon as I got home. Not eating, she said, was not a good idea at all. Not drinking was even worse. I thought, okay then; and thanks, but let me try something first.

I thought to myself that I just couldn't go back to a hospital right now. I had just gotten out of the hospital with pneumonia. I was depressed thinking how much worse my health was bound to get as the chemotherapy treatments continued, and this was only my second dose. Unless I began to use my head I would find myself in the hospital more often than I cared to think about. I had five more months of it to go, and began to wonder if I really could make it through until the end of the treatments in August.

Use your head girl, I thought. Think of something fast or you'll be in the working end of a hospital bed before morning. I took the only way out I could think of. Rats!

I took the next exit and bought a kid's size hamburger at the first fast-food restaurant I came to. I felt hungry, somewhat hungry anyway. But, the thought of swallowing anything just about brought me to defeat. Here goes nothing, I thought. I had another 180 miles of driving before I got home and it took me the rest of the trip to get that lousy hamburger down. But, I ate it all. After drinking as much Maalox as I could I went straight to bed when I got home. Maalox didn't help much, but I thought it was better than nothing.

The next morning I began to cook. I didn't stop cooking until I had four full-course meals prepared and stored in the refrigerator. With that taken care of, I hit the couch again in complete exhaustion. When I woke up, I began to eat while wishing I didn't have to. I ate until I just couldn't cram down another bite. I hated, even resented, every bite I had to swallow. You know how it is though. You will do whatever it takes.

In the next day or two the burning subsided a bit. I got back into drinking my water. I drank enough water to sink a battle ship, which gave me something to do (running back and forth to the bathroom). Through all of this my esophagus gave me trouble to be sure, but not so much that I couldn't eat in order to stay out of the hospital. It was very uncomfortable, but I learned you could do things that need to be done if you try hard enough. What I did had little to do with being brave, but had everything to do with staying alive. I found that to be a profound difference.

Although I didn't go to the hospital, it all worked out anyway. However, if I couldn't have eaten, I would have gone to the ER. I skinned out of that one by a thin hair. I chalked up another 'at-a-girl'. This cancer just had to go, that's all there was to it!

The two weeks without chemotherapy helped my esophagus calm down a bit more. Eating wasn't so terribly uncomfortable, although I was extremely careful about what and when I ate, and I took the rest of Dale's OTC Prolosec. Did the Prolosec help? I guess I can't really say. If it didn't help me in a physical way, I'm sure it helped me in an emotional way. In the end I guess I believe it helped.

As the days worn on I considered my condition and what lay ahead. You know how you feel when you have the flu? How you can't remember ever feeling well, and how you think you'll never feel well again? That was me. I really did wonder if I would ever feel healthy again. However, I did feel in much better shape as I left for my next treatment. My attitude was one of, "Here we go again". I wondered what new and amazing malady would rear its ugly head this time around?

Before my next treatment I was given my usual blood test upon arrival at the cancer center. The results showed that my neutrophils were in the proverbial tank. They were so low, in fact, that I didn't take a treatment that day. I wouldn't take my third treatment until my blood counts regained stability. However, some how, the doctor felt that the cancer had stopped its forward motion. I had only two treatments behind me, so I was surprised to hear that... but very happy. I asked him what I could do to get my neutrophils up again, as I was afraid I had caused the problem when I couldn't eat. He told me it wasn't my fault, that the chemotherapy was to blame. As I wasn't allowed vitamins and supplements while taking chemotherapy, all I could do was eat. So, I ate... again...Rats!

I had four weeks without chemotherapy this time, which I hoped would give my body a well-deserved rest from the drugs. During that time, however, I was in and out of the emergency room or the doctor's office a few times to ward off pneumonia and for a severe infection whose cause is still a mystery to me. One of the problems that sent me to the emergency room again was pounding heart palpitations.

I was running the vacuum over the kitchen floor at home when the palpitations hit. They came on suddenly, caught me by surprise, and scared me to death. Remembering that the port carried the chemo drugs uncomfortably close to my heart, the possibility of a heart attack crossed my mind. However, I didn't feel any other symptom that I thought should accompany a heart attack. Although, I wasn't sure what those other symptoms should be. I didn't know what to do, but knew I didn't want to be the dummy that called 911 and have it be a false alarm. Likely, that wasn't the smartest decision I've ever made, but I really didn't know what was causing the palpitations.

Even though I didn't know the best way to handle this whole thing I thought that, maybe, if I just lay down, the palpations would subside. So, I lay down on the couch and waited for the pounding to stop. Well...nothing stopped. I lay there for about five minutes with my heart pounding hard enough to make my head feel like it was rocking. Then, my chest began to hurt a little more than I thought it should, and my color turned a little too gray. It was time to get help. I didn't think that driving myself to the hospital this time would be such a good idea. If I passed out I could cause an accident. I didn't want to get stuck out in the boonies with no help either, nor did I want to cause injury to someone else. Lastly, I couldn't afford to wreak another car. So, I began to call friends. As luck would have it no one was home, so I couldn't get in touch with anyone. Then I remembered Kam.

I called Kam, a friend of mine, and asked if she would run me up to the hospital. Kam is one of those people who you've known your entire life even if you've just met her. She is the owner of the restaurant where Dale and I were when Dale died. I believe it nearly broke her heart when she saw Dale lying on the floor that Sunday morning. In a very determined voice she promised to be 'right there'!

I didn't feel that tidying up nor taking care of the vacuum was of any particular importance, so I let it lay on the floor where I dropped it. When Kam arrived she took a look at me and said, "You look like s***" (Well, she didn't think I looked so good). That's Kam, though. When a thought comes to her mind it's out of her mouth and on its way to your ear in a veritable flash. For her, she simply says what's on her mind, she's not the least bit rude about it; it's just something that needs to be said...so...she says it. Her comment sort of struck me funny. It wasn't intended as criticism, it was an observation born of considerable concern. I acknowledged that she was likely right, and she suggested that we needed to get going.

We got going! By that time of night our single traffic light was blinking yellow when we zoomed under it. Try to conjure a mental picture of a bunch of teenaged boys that have been let loose in a go-cart. Now you've got the picture! It's good that our local city police help roll up the sidewalks after dark, then go home to watch Jeopardy on television. Otherwise, things could have gotten very interesting very quickly. All that was on her mind was to get help. She wasn't so sure whether my heart was about to cave in or not, and CPR wasn't something she had planned for that evening.

Actually it was one of those incidences in life where you're sure you shouldn't be laughing inside...but you are. I mean, I was trying not to, and laughing certainly didn't occur to her. The event wasn't funny at all, but the situation seemed funny to me. However, it didn't take long for the humor to ebb.

We were less than ten minutes from the hospital when the palpations abruptly stopped. I asked her to take me back home thinking I couldn't be having a heart attack or I would have been getting worse instead of better. It didn't appear to me that she thought going back home was a good idea, but she finally agreed. It's good that I did go home though. When I arrived back home I found, in my haste, I had left eggs boiling on the stove. Do you sometimes wonder why bad things (like house fires) happen to good people? It's because, sometimes, good people do stupid things. That would be me.

By this time I was getting really very weary of traumas. I knew things couldn't, and wouldn't come close to being normal again for a very long time. I knew I had to 'keep going' as there was no other choice. But, I was getting very tired of it all. I let the vacuum lay on the kitchen floor thinking I could take care of it in the morning. Tomorrow was another day, and I'd had enough. I just flopped down on the couch and went to sleep.

Nothing happened after I got home, nor for the rest of the night. The following morning the palpations began again while I was getting out of the shower. Not again...! I tried lying down again, and again, it did no good. This time I called Reg, made sure nothing was left cooking on the stove, and got ready to go to the hospital.

He and his wife and I were on our way to the hospital when the palpitations stopped again. This time I wanted to know what the heck was going on. Furthermore, I didn't entertain the idea that Reg would have taken be back home anyway, so we continued on to the hospital. After being examined in the emergency room, I was admitted.

I ended up in the hospital over night that time. I was monitored all night and into the next morning. Because I couldn't be monitored during the palpitations though, the testing and monitoring showed nothing. So, the doctor scheduled a chemically induced stress test for the following Monday. I went home thinking that my heart must be in pretty good shape to take a beating like that and come out of it like nothing had happened. At least something was still working like it should.

While all of this was taking place, Bryan (the friend with the food route) stopped by to see how I was. Obviously, he didn't get a response when he knocked on the door, and he couldn't get in to see if I was lying dead somewhere, but he did see the vacuum lying in the kitchen. He took that as a crystal clear indication that all was not well in the Hulliberger house. Well, that started a chain of events that caused some emotional commotion among my friends. He called one of them after another to see if they knew where I was; they didn't know. They called other friends to check on my whereabouts, and the next person did the same. Pretty soon an alarmed concern for my welfare was in full bloom. Eventually, they got in touch with Chuck and Joan who had a key. My home was frisked, but they found nothing (obviously).

They must have called Reg after he got home, because they learned I was in the hospital. When I got home the next day I found a note lying on the bar. It was direct, short, and to the point. "If you want to live through this…let us know when something happens". Tears welled. There was a mountain of love and concern in that note. Albeit, between the lines. The next day, bright and early, Bryan was there with nails, a hammer, and a white board. He had a marker pencil with a little sticky thing to hold the marker to the board that was attached to the side panel of my entrance door. I was given instructions for its use.

After leaving a detailed message for my friends on my new white board, I kept my appointment for the stress test that Monday morning. I was lying on a gurney, of sorts, waiting for the technician to get the stress test underway. She proved to be a grouch, and muttered that I must be a lazy one because I hadn't been scheduled for the regular treadmill stress test. I took her comment as a bit of a challenge, and asked her what she had been doing for the past four months. When she didn't answer I told her I was a terminal cancer patient who didn't have the strength for the treadmill.

Okay, maybe I didn't know if I had the strength for the treadmill or not, but she didn't know that either. She should have kept her thoughts to herself. I didn't much care whether she thought I was a 'lazy one' or not. I thought that she was either having a bad day, or her personality made her more competent to work in a library. You know...some place where she had to be *quiet*. Either way, she was busy trying to take her foot out of her mouth, so I didn't have verbal comments from her throughout the rest of the test.

Just a side note here...the next stress test I take will be on the treadmill if at all possible. I'm not fond of what the chemicals do. One minute I felt just fine, and the next minute I was back into the pounding heart palpations again. I'll never know for a certain fact, but I think the tech could have gotten a subversive pleasure out of my discomfort. Or, it could have been that I was just in a very bad mood. Either way, we were both enjoying ourselves.

I found out months later that the palpitations were probably caused from panic attacks, (go figure). I also found out that I had to get them stopped as quickly as I could. There is some danger in allowing your heart to beat that hard and that fast for any length of time. I have a bottle of Xanax in my purse...just in case.

After I got home from the stress test I began to tally the good and not so good effects that the chemo treatments were having on my body. The nausea wasn't a problem like I'd heard it could be, likely due to the million-dollar nausea pills I was given. But, I was getting pretty weak and plenty tired. The toenail of my large toe, right foot, was showing signs of coming off, and did. However, the rest of my nails seemed to be doing okay, but they all hurt, as did my fingernails. My appetite was a dieter's dream; I just wasn't hungry and actually dreaded eating anything. I slept most of the day and night, and my hair began to take on all the qualities of dead straw. My skin didn't look so good. I looked sick even when I didn't feel sick. All in all, I just felt rotten, and felt I was going downhill from there. It was apparent that the chemotherapy drugs were surely showing their bad side in force. However, I was still alive, which weighs heavily on the plus side of drugs. And, I had to remember that the chemotherapy drugs had stopped the forward motion of the cancer. That's a very big plus in my vocabulary.

# Protocel ®

It was now mid April of 2006. I had just arrived at my brother house, and was mentally getting ready for another chemo treatment that was scheduled for the next day. Karla gave me a letter that had been sent from my cousin, Joanne, in Pennsylvania. In the letter, Joanne told me about a natural product called Protocel®. She suggested that I try it. I nearly dismissed the information in the letter, and would have if she hadn't been a retired registered nurse. But, it was when she wrote that my other cousin's husband, Joe, was using Protocel® for his lung cancer, and with a great amount of success, that stirred my curiosity enough to take another look. I thought of Joe as having a similar outlook on such matters as I did. I knew Joe, and knew he wouldn't put his trust in Protocel®, or anything else for that matter, without first believing that it could work. I have always considered myself an open-minded skeptic, and now my skepticism, along with my curiosity, was working overtime.

However, I had a good doctor, and I was getting the help I didn't think I was going to get, so why rock the boat? Then again, I knew that I needed more help with the cancer than the chemotherapy could offer, so my skepticism took a backseat to my curiosity.

While I was thinking all of this over I was reminded that any doctor who dealt with my prognosis had the same answer. Chemotherapy would never completely get rid of the cancer, so the most I was gaining with chemotherapy treatments was a little more time. I was glad to get more time, but it was the promise of impending death that I was thinking about now. Although I was getting help, in the end, it wouldn't be enough. I was still going to die sooner than I thought I should. Dying was just going to take a little longer, and I wanted to live. There had to be a way, and Protocel® could very well be the answer. Skepticism and curiosity took a backseat to hope.

While reading all the information I could find on Protocel® I found that Protocel® isn't supposed to work well with some conventional treatments and/or chemotherapy drugs. However, there are exceptions. 5-FU and radiation are examples of two of those exceptions. 5-FU is considered an anti-metabolic chemotherapy and works well with Protocel®. The good news I found was that Protocel® is non-invasive, and it can be taken for the rest of your life, if you choose, without harm. I had learned the hard way that chemotherapy drugs will cause physical problems almost from the beginning, remembering though that chemotherapy was the reason I was still alive. Very sick...but still alive.

There were two other chemo drugs that I was taking that weren't supposed to work well with Protocel®. However, I was thinking that those drugs were just going to have to make room, because Protocel® began to look pretty good to me.

While I was researching Protocel® I began to feel hope stir in my soul. I read what it did, but I still didn't have an understanding about how it accomplished its end result. I wanted to know; I wanted to reason it out, how Protocel®

actually killed cancer cells. Knowing how it worked would help me believe. Belief would feed my hope and courage. Hope and courage would help me fight. I needed all the tools I could get my hands wrapped around. So, I looked on.

I found Ty Bollinger's book *Cancer: Step Outside the Box* where I found all the information I had hoped to find. Here is what I learned. Here is were I found my hope and courage. Read on in faith...

## Cell Biology: 101

Imagine your body is a country and the cells are it citizens. In order for the country to be strong, its citizens must have various jobs, proper tools to do their jobs, proper nutrition to stay healthy, a transportation system, a communication system, a waste disposal system, a safe place to rest, and protection from toxins who wish to do them harm. We need to provide our cells with all of these requirements.

We have all different types of cells, and they all have a brain that is called the nucleus. Red blood cells are the only cells in our body that do not have a nucleus. All others do.

Then there is the cell membrane, or the skin and is made of protein molecules. Some of these proteins act like a "name tag" to identify the type of call, while other proteins act as a door to the cell. Next is the cell fiber, which could be called the scaffolding; and could be view as the muscles of the cell, which helps the cells expand and contract into different shapes. Inside all of this are *organelles*. They are like "little organs," and each of them has a specific function.

Healthy cells are called "aerobic, meaning that they function properly in the presence of sufficient oxygen. Healthy cells 'burn' oxygen and glucose (blood sugar) to produce something that is called "adenosine triphosphate – or ATP which is the energy current of the cells. All of this is called...aerobic respiration. This cycle of creating energy is called the Krebs cycle and takes place in the inner and outer membranes (the *mitochondria*).

ATP is composed of three phosphates. Breaking the bond between the second and third phosphate releases the energy to power virtually all cellular processes. Each of our 60 trillion cells consumes and regenerates 12 million molecules of ATP a day. Amazing. But, without ATP our cells couldn't live.

## Foreign Invaders

When foreign invaders enter the body, our immune system comes to the rescue. The immune system is a collection of cells, chemical messengers, and proteins that work together to protect the body from potential harm. The immune systems leukocytes (white blood cells) are our bodies #1 defense. There are two main subgroups of leukocytes. Polymorphonoclear and monoculear. Monocytes ingest dead or damaged cells and provide defenses against many infectious organisms.

It takes several days - to weeks - for lymphocytes to recognize and attack a new foreign substance. The main lymphocyte sub-types are B-cells, T-cells, and NK (Natural Killer) cells.

## Aerobic vs. Anaerobic Respiration

Remember that the cycle of creating energy is called the Krebs cycle and takes place in the mitochondria. Cells typically create energy via a process known as aerobic respiration (i.e. "with oxygen). However, if something happens to alter this cycle then the cell is damaged for the lack of its ability to produce ATP. Since, the Krebs cycle has been disrupted, the cells have no energy, and we have a serious problem because the cell doesn't have enough oxygen for it to breathe.

Now, we have an anaerobic cell to contend with. Since there isn't enough oxygen for the cell to breathe, it changes to an anaerobic cell respiration-type to survive (i.e. "without oxygen").

Dr. David Gregg says, "Cancer does not cause cells to turn anaerobic, but rather it is stabilized anaerobic respiration that is the single cause (or essential requirement) that turns the normal calls that depend on aerobic respiration into cancer cells. (www.krysalis.net)

The cell stops breathing oxygen and start fermenting glucose (sugar) to make energy. When that takes place the outside of the cell wall becomes coated with a dense layer of protein and inhibits oxygen from getting into the cell. The protein inhibits the white blood cells from doing their job of attacking and destroying invaders...including cancer cells.

Because anaerobic cells must work harder to survive they cause a 'severe' drain on the body. Think of it this way...

In order for a cancer cell to obtain the same energy as a normal cell it must metabolize at least 18 times more glucose than a normal 'aerobic' cell. Now do you see why we should pay particular attention to the phrase "cancer loves sugar"?

A cancer cell grows indefinitely and without order in an acidic and low Oxygen environment. Over coming cancer is a process of reversing the conditions that allowed the cancer to develop.

For more information on this subject and pH balance, read Ty Bollinger's book *Cancer: Step Outside the Box.* Available at Amazon.com.

## Non-Toxic Protocel

Jim Sheridan, a devout Christian, created Protocel. The first formula created was called Entelev, which, in Greek means "entelechy" (that part of man known only to God). It was eventually renamed "cancel", and is currently sold as Protocel.

## What Protocel® is and how it works

It is the world's most effective free radical scavenger (antioxidant). It is designed to specifically target anaerobic cells (i.e. cancer) by interfering with the production of ATP energy in all the body's cells. It reduces the 'voltage' in each cell by 10 to 20 percent.

The slight reduction in voltage causes anaerobic cancer cells to shift downward to a point below the minimum that they need to remain in tact, thus the cells basically self-destruct and break apart, or "lyse" into harmless proteins. The healthy cells of the body typically have such a high normal voltage that the slight reduction in voltage caused by Protocel® does not harm them.

The scientific basis for Protocel® is to place a long-term drain of energy power on cancer cells. The long-term drain of power causes the cell to slowly loose its respiratory abilities. As long as there is a drain of power the inhibition of respiratory ability continues until the cell reaches the 'critical point' in its life. One of the chemicals in the body, catechol, is taken advantage of by Protocel. Catechol forces the cell further down to the point where the body recognizes it as 'bad', then attacks the weakened anaerobic cell and disposes of it.

Cancer cells may become M.D.R. (Multiple-drug Resistant). In other words...if cancer cells mutate, then you would be wise to add Paw Paw as a supplement. Paw Paw will not only kill the M.D.R. cells, it will also enhance the effectiveness of Protocel in other ways.

The combination of Paw Paw with Protocel® is a powerful "cancer-fighting" cocktail. In order to maximize the effectiveness of this cocktail, they should be taken every 6 hours, on the hour, 24 hours a day, and 7 days a week. To be safe, it is recommended that vitamin C and Vitamin E be eliminated as supplements since these antioxidants increase the ATP, thus would negate the effectiveness of Protocel and Paw Paw.

So...

- Protocel is the world's most effective free radical scavenger (antioxidant).
- Designed to target anaerobic cells by interfering with the production of ATP energy (lowers the cells voltage [energy]).
- Lowers the voltage by 10% to 20% and the anaerobic cell dies.
- When the anaerobic cell dies...the cancer cell dies.

I am in debt to Ty Bollinger for all of his tireless research, as his knowledge became my hope. His information became an ingredient in the mix that could save my life, and it can save yours. Buy his book and read it. You won't be sorry you did.

I went to the Internet again and found the website www. *outsmartyourcancer.com*, and read the articles I found there. I sent for and read the book *Out Smart Your Cancer;* authored by Tanya Harter Pierce. In her book I read a lot of testimonials from former cancer patients who had found complete success with Protocel®. Not just more time...complete success! Not much was said about combining Protocel® with chemo-therapy though, so I was somewhat concerned about that. However, my doctor at Karmanos had told me earlier that 48 hours after the needle that delivered the chemo drugs was pulled, the chemotherapy drugs were no longer active. So... that meant that my body would have eleven days between treatments without the benefit of any cancer-killing therapy.

There would be no drug interaction with the cancer. Unless, that is, I began taking the Protocel®.

I could do a little experimenting, I thought. What could it hurt…what did I have to loose? My death was a predicted reality. That was a 'cause and effect' I felt I knew something about. So, what harm would it do to give it a try? What's the worst that could happen, I could die? Between the cancer and the chemotherapy I was well on my way to that particular destination anyway. Adding a new bullet to this war on cancer seemed like a good idea to me. And, this was a bullet void of 'friendly fire'. It would destroy only the enemy. That thought brought jubilation bubbling to the surface.

I believed that Protocel® really could help me. So, I sent for it. However, it sat on my kitchen counter, and I stared at it for a week wondering what to do (I seem to have a gift for confounding myself). Confusion loves company, and I was great company. Finally, on April 21st of 2006 I threw concern to the wind and began taking the Protocel®.

## What a difference!

I don't know exactly when the transformation took place, but it wasn't long, and it was *astounding* to say the least. Before I began taking Protocel® I was weak, sickly, weary, and my blood counts weren't anything to write home about. I ate just to stay out of the hospital, and feeling sick all the time did nothing to boost my emotions.

Then, one day I realized, holy cow! I feel better! I looked in the mirror and realized that I didn't look quite so 'dead'. My hair still looked as though I needed a bailer rather than a comb, but that didn't worry me. Even the acid reflux was almost completely gone, and that all by itself made Protocel® worth its weight in pure gold! My energy was increasing, and I didn't feel like I had to spend so much time in bed. I began to think of food as a good thing again. And, my overall feeling of well-being was improving. I wondered what other good things were going on inside my body that I couldn't see.

Do you know what though? When the Protocel® revelation became apparent to me I wasn't thinking about whether or not it was killing my cancer. At that point in time I was consumed by feelings of utter ecstasy because I felt good again. I began to think about getting out of bed in the morning in a positive way. Real belief in my ability to function began to take root. I could wonder about the cancer-killing ability of Protocel® after I got used to the reaction of feeling close to normal again. To say that I was surprised to find that Protocel® could make that dramatic a difference in my emotional and physical health was, at the very least, an understatement.

I had been taking Protocel® for approximately three weeks and wondered if it was interfering in any way with my conventional treatments. Thinking about it now, I guess that the only thing that had the ability to interfere with chemotherapy drugs would be a small dose of real battery acid. There's no battery acid in Protocel®, so I guessed that I was safe. I thought that three weeks was long enough for a problem with the chemotherapy/Protocel® mix to show up if it was going to. I would find out soon, as the blood labs would tell me what was happening on my next treatment day.

I was elated when, at my next treatment, I found the lab results showed my blood counts were back in the normal range. I was amazed all over again, and I was just plain grateful. The doctor was surprised with the results too, as I'm sure that he hadn't expected much, if any, improvement at all.

I didn't tell my doctor about the Protocel®. I had learned that oncologists have no belief or patience in anything that is labeled natural and/or 'drugless'. Usually I have to be clunked over the head just once before I learn a lesson, and this was one of those times. Way back in December, I had tried to discuss natural supplements with an oncologist for the very last time. If my doctor was curious and wanted to know if I was doing something out of his normal routine for therapy, then he would ask. Otherwise, he would remain unaware. I wasn't in the mood to have my self-esteem slapped around again. That wasn't anything against my good doctor; it was simply self-defense on my part. I had seen enough good results in the last month to make me truly believe that I needed the Protocel® to get healthy again. Therefore, I wouldn't have stopped taking it even if the doctor suggested that I did. So, why stir up a rat's nest when I didn't have to. That may not have been the best logic, but it's the only logic that registered with me at the time.

In hindsight, I probably should have told the doctor about my Protocel®. Without me confessing the Protocel® he had no way of knowing that the chemo drugs weren't totally responsible for the improvements. Would he have upped the chemotherapy drug dosage thinking that more was better? Good grief! Just thinking about adding more chemo to the 51 hours I was already taking makes me shiver. I'm thinking that because my condition was improving so quickly, and knowing how bad the cancer was in the beginning; he must have guessed that I was doing something other than his regi-ment. I guess that's a reasonable assumption, so I'll just leave it that way. Finally, I actually had a rational thought. About time!

# PICC Line

By now the port site was in pretty bad condition because of the infection, and had to be removed. I had given the infection a lot of thought. I could think of only two reasons why the site infected in the first place. I wondered if it could be that my immune system couldn't fight off the infection because of the cancer and the chemotherapy drugs that I was taking. That didn't make a lot of sense to me because my blood counts were now in the normal range. I guessed that if my blood counts were normal then my immune system should have been able get the port site healthy. Also, the site became infected even before I began taking the chemotherapy, so it had to be the cancer, or something else completely.

Then, I'd found out there was a small amount of metal in the type of port that was used. That, for me, was the likely cause. I can't wear pierced earrings no matter how expensive they are, as my ears will become infected almost immediately. Metal that pierces any part of my body, and remains like pierced earrings do, just doesn't work. I'd never dreamed of having a nose ring, so body metal was not much of a concern until the port. It was decided that the port would have to be removed and a PICC line would be used in its place.

The difference between the port and the PICC line, other than position, is longevity. It's felt that a PICC line will infect more quickly than a port. However, that was the only other solution. I hoped that the PICC line would outlast my need for it.

So, an appointment to take out the port and insert the PICC line was set up. Again, Duane took me to the hospital to have this procedure taken care of. Again, I was given the option of being put to sleep, or they could administer the local anesthetic. I bounced that offer around for a hasty minute before I jumped all over it. The port would have to be removed, and the PICC line inserted. I wasn't feeling so brave this time, nor I did I feel a great need to be awake for it. There would be a two-hour wait in the hospital after I awoke, but I didn't care. I was prepped, given a shot, and the world went away.

When I awoke the procedure was over and I found that everything went well. I had a brand new PICC line that was positioned in the inside of my right upper arm. Now I wanted to leave the hospital, but there was that blasted two-hour wait.

I could still be a whinny woman when I needed to be (batting your eyelashes after your sixtieth birthday has very little impact), so I was able to talk the doctor into letting me go before the two-hour wait was up. I was going right to the cancer clinic for another treatment anyway, and I could be monitored there just as easily as in the hospital. No one likes a whiner, so he reluctantly released me; or, maybe happily got rid of me. Either way, I got the distinct impression he felt that his day would improve when mine did. Duane and I left for my treatment. I had a very strong feeling that the PICC line would do its job, and I decided that I wasn't going to worry about it. I had my chemotherapy treatment that day, and everything went just fine.

I continued to take the chemotherapy drugs along with the Protocel®, and I continued to feel good. My doctor seemed pleased with my progress. In fact, during one of my treatments he came to my chemo booth to talk with me, and he actually gave me a high-five. Right after the high-five he reminded me that, although I was doing better than expected, I shouldn't be surprised if I took a turn for the worse. I thought how I wished he had kept that to himself. I wanted to tell him that I would ask when I wanted to be reminded that I was still going to die. Until then, please let me have my hope. Tomorrow had always taken care of itself, and I had no reason to believe that had changed.

There is no doubt he had no intentions of hurting me with his words, but his words did hurt. It took another two or three days of talking to myself to get my "hope meter" back up where it belonged. In his defense, his experience had told him that I was still dying, that there still was no hope. Likely he didn't want me to get my hopes high just to have them dashed in the end. Like I said, his intent wasn't to hurt me. Cancer is tough on everyone.

The Protocel® was still new to me, so I wondered if it really would get rid of the cancer completely. Inasmuch, I had a long way to go, and my disposition had greatly improved, I felt good. I decided that if I could feel this good until the day I died then it had been worth any conceived risk involved in taking it. It hadn't weakened any of my chemotherapy drugs as far as I could see, and it didn't appear that the drugs had dampened the effects of the Protocel® much either. There was no doubt, as far as I was concerned, that I had made the right decision.

Then, sometime in May, something happened that I hadn't expected. I noticed hard bumps were beginning to appear under the skin of my left arm, and they itched like crazy. Each day more bumps appeared until my arm was covered.

Finally, I called Dr. Bell (the bio chemist) and asked him what could be the cause.

Listen to this....

He said, "Elaine, you're killing the cancer too fast. Your liver is overwhelmed by the toxins (dead cancer cells), and is storing the toxins in the lymph nodes of your arm until it can better handle them". "All you have to do is quit taking Protocel® for three days and drink a lot of water. The rash will go away".

Killing cancer too fast? Are you kidding? You couldn't kill cancer too fast as far as I was concerned. If I needed another problem that's the one I would have picked, hands down! My liver, however, had problems of its own. It was fighting its own tumor, plus all the extra toxins that were coming its way. It was screaming, "Enough already!"

I couldn't ignore Dr. Bell's advice, and didn't want to labor my liver anymore than I already had. I decided to quit taking Protocel® for a full week and give my liver a real break. However, after being off Protocel® for three days I began to feel really sick and weak again. The reflux problem was returning, and all I wanted to do was lay in bed. Eating wasn't a priority, and my feelings of well being turned to gloom again. On the fourth day I started back on the Protocel® and began to feel better almost immediately. Just as Dr. Bell promised the bumps disappeared, and they never returned. Killing cancer to fast? That's a scenario I hadn't thought of!

I took that whole episode with the rash as proof positive that the Protocel® was truly killing a ton of cancer cell. Otherwise the bumps wouldn't have disappeared when I stopped the Protocel® for three days. Also, reverting from feeling so lousy while off the Protocel® to feeling healthy again so quickly after getting back on it is a testament to Protocel's® ability to enhance my immune system. At least that's the way I saw it.

It's true that the chemotherapy drugs stopped my cancer's forward growth. It's also true that the chemo drugs had the capability to inhibit my body's ability to recover completely. I didn't want to trade dying of cancer to dying of chemotherapy drugs. However, I really didn't want to stop the chemo because my cancer was so extensive. I still felt I needed all the help I could get my hands on. After all my chemo treatments were done, and it had killed all the cancer it was able to kill; then, I thought the Protocel® could finish off the rest of the cancer on its own. That was my plan. I would have to wait to see if it worked.

All that really mattered to me then was that I was getting better, and I was feeling better. Right then, all I knew was that it wasn't enough just to be alive. I wanted to be alive with the quality of life that we all want. That's what I felt the Protocel® was doing for to me, where chemotherapy was helping, but only offered more time. It was my prayer that Protocel® would see me all the way through. So, I just kept going.

## Another CT Scan

It was now the end of May, and I had undergone six chemotherapy treatments. It was time for the second CT scan in Detroit. The CT scan was taken during my off-week from chemo, so I wouldn't know how things were going until I returned for my next treatment date.

I drove home after my treatment, like always. I tried to keep my mind off the results of the CT scan, and just let one day dissolve into the next like always. But what the test results would show was always right there under the surface of my 'what if' thinking. I was having a controlled anxiety attack (what fun), but I got through it just fine.

When the treatment day arrived the doctor was about to give me the results of the CT scan. I held my breath. I'm not kidding; I literally held my breath.

The news was good. The news was *very* good! The tumors were beginning to reduce in size! Thank you God! Thank you Doctors! And, thank you Protocel®! I didn't expect it, I'm not sure I believed it, but it was real. The combination of chemotherapy and Protocel® were actually killing the cancer! And, they were doing it more quickly than anyone would have ever guessed. All I had heard for the last six months was that I was going to die… no matter what. Maybe, just maybe, my prognosis was turning around. I felt the sort of hope you can feel, hear, and taste as much as recognize. It was my emotional turning point. Inhibitions were all that prevented me from dancing a jig!

However, it seemed to me that every time I had a good report, like this one, the doctor reminded me that, although I had a positive report this time, the next report could very well be bad. I came to label that part of my treatments as "reports from the death squad". It could be argued that he had a good reason for his reminders of impending death, but I haven't decided yet what that could be. Maybe it's seeing the dashed hopes of a cancer patient, instead of death, that some oncologists can't deal with. All I know is that this doctor was nearly as happy with the results of the CT scan as I was. And, it was obvious that he hadn't expected that much of an improvement that quickly…maybe not at all.

It was time for some good news, and as for me, I was basking in the news! I took the good report as positive and hopeful, and decided that I wouldn't remain rooted in fear. No one knew better than I did that the road ahead promised to be a long one. But, make no mistake…hope smoothes out the bumps like no medicine can. Again, I don't believe my doctor was trying to hurt me in any way. However, I didn't understand his need for the reminders either, and I guess I still don't.

I would like to be able to say that I always acted in a congenial and grateful way, but the truth is I didn't always do that. Most days I was just fine, then there were the days where I was quiet, unsociable and moody. I can get pretty cranky. The nurses and volunteers at the center had to muster up their own understanding and patience where I was concerned, just as much as I had to understand some of the things they did or said. After ministering help to a room full of people like me it's a wonder they found pleasure in their work at all. They deserve a tremendous amount of praise, and I don't think they get a lot of that sort of thing. Treating cancer isn't a good experience for anyone.

After I got the good news I had a deep-rooted urge to take this report back up North, where my arrogant surgeon was, and ask him how many people he had let die. No, I didn't do that. If this report would matter to him, then in the beginning, *I* would have mattered to him. The only thing that would change his attitude would be for him to find himself in his patient's shoes. God forbid that happens, even to him. The jerk!

My outlook and energy improved, and my treatment routine continued. The day before my treatment I drove to Monroe and stayed overnight with Duane and Karla. They're both great people and I enjoyed being with them. Duane can be a real comic, and so I found myself laughing a lot. Karla is a good lady who welcomed me in her home and helped me as much as she could. She took me in even though she is suffering with heart problems. Duane took off work to take care of me. Okay, you can guess what that meant to me. Sometimes angels don't have wings; sometimes they look a lot like family.

I really would have liked to see my son, Randy, though; and wished I could fly to Georgia, or he could fly to Michigan for a day or two. His job and my treatments got in the way of that reunion for a while yet. But, that would soon change

# The Vacation

Because Randy lived three states away he couldn't do as much for me as he would have liked. But, he gave me as much long distance support as he could. As soon as he was able he and his family came home for three days and took me to one of my treatments. Cancer or no cancer, we had a good time. We didn't do anything special for those three days, but we enjoyed the time we had together, and I can tell you we were happy to have the chance to be together.

Later, in June, he was able to get enough vacation time to take me on a motorcycle trip to Northern Michigan. A vacation!! I was ready for that!

Randy came home again, but this time on his motorcycle. He brought his wife's motorcycle clothing and helmet for me to wear on our trip. I tried them on, the clothing fit, and the vacation was underway! It was the first recreation I had been involved in for well over a year, and I was looking forward to doing something 'normal'. It was summer time, the weather was good, and we were on our way.

We stayed in a motel with a view of the Mackinac Bridge. The bridge is quite a sight during the day, but it's almost surreal at night. The first day we just poked around, took pictures, and otherwise just enjoyed the scenery. We decided to drive across the bridge on the second day to see the Soo Locks.

Crossing the Mackinac Bridge on a motorcycle on the way over was a real event for me. But, crossing back was an event for both of us. The wind was gusting and whipping the bike quite a bit. It wasn't too bad most of the time, as Randy kept good control. We had to lean into the wind, but when we passed a pylon the bike would abruptly straighten.

He had to compensate the weight shift for both of us the first couple of times, as I wasn't used to that sort of thing. It doesn't take long to learn though.

I'm sure neither of us expected to be plummeted over the rail, but the ride did capture our attention. I wasn't frightened at all, but was glad I didn't have a scientific understanding of the effects that wind had on motorcycle tires, bridge grating, and weight shift. Stupidity is sometimes a veritable blessing.. There were other bikes having the same problem that we were, but I don't think there was any real danger for any of us, and soon we were all off the bridge and on solid ground once more. What a day! What fun!

I was so glad to be with Randy...my mind went back to when Randy was a baby using his crib for a trampoline. When he used the cast on his broken arm for a ball bat, and when he put his arm around my shoulder in front of his high school friends. Time and miles had kept us at a distance for quite a few years. But, all those years and all that distance weren't important anymore. Our vacation came to an end, but we truly enjoyed the time we had together. My mind was away from cancer and problems in general, and we had a lot of fun in those three days.

## The Doll

I had another treatment scheduled for the Tuesday following our vacation. While taking this treatment at the center a lady came to see me at my chemo booth. She asked if I would like to make a doll. A doll? Why not, I thought.

This is how it works. You write something you want to do, or something you want to change in your life on a piece of paper. You roll the message to yourself up in a ball. That ball of paper is covered with fabric and used as the doll's head. Then, using only fabric and a hot-glue gun, the rest of the doll is constructed. It belongs to you. It is a constant reminder that there will be a tomorrow. I am still touched just thinking about the lady and the doll. I keep it on my bookshelves where I can see it every day.

The Protocel® was keeping my blood counts in the normal range, so I missed no more chemo treatments. And, my doctors and nurses were doing their best.

Duane and Karla took me out to dinner once in a while on the days I was with them. We went to the lake, shopped, and did little fun things like that. I couldn't get Duane to go back to work though. He has his own business, so he wasn't in danger of being fired, but he was losing a ton of business because of my cancer. I was so dependent on him. He said he would go back to work when I was well. God will bless him.

While I was at home my friends stopped in just to chat and to assure themselves that I was doing okay. Some would e-mail me, and some would give me a phone call. Others would stop by so I could ride with them as they did their errands, just for the company. I didn't go fishing when I had the chance, didn't go to the movies, or any social event for that matter. I wasn't used to doing those sorts of things without Dale yet and felt more like the fifth-wheel than I should have. Along with the people in my life, and putting all the cancer and the effects of the chemotherapy aside...I was doing pretty darn good. Sure, I had my unhappy days, and, there were even moments when I didn't think I was going to make it. I guess I don't think feelings like I've described are so very unusual considering the issues I was facing. But, all things considered, I really was doing okay.

I would have found it very interesting to discuss days like those with someone who had gone through similar times. I would have liked to know how they defended themselves against their depressed days, and frightful moments. I wonder how they began to build a different kind of life? It didn't seem to be the overall picture of a future I was looking at during those times. It was the time lapse between one minute and the next that held my attention. I know it would have been a source of comfort to be able to talk with someone who had been where I found myself at that time in my life. However, somehow I learned that I could, and I would go on. My friends and family gave me hope, laughter, and grit. What more could I expect, or ask, under the circumstances. I really was doing just fine.

Also, I had found a haven for Bubba, as well. Shawn and Angie have three children, and live out in the country where Bubba could play with their kids and run as much as he liked. To Dale and me, Shawn and Angie were like our own children. Bubba is a happy camper.

## June's CT Scan

Another CT scan was taken in June, which showed the tumors were still reducing in size. Each time positive test reports came back my thoughts went back to the beginning. If Duane and Karla hadn't told me about the doctors in Detroit, and if Joanne hadn't told me about Protocel®, I could very well have been dead by now. Instead, I was reading another positive report. I took things one day at a time, but there were times when I couldn't help thinking how desperate things were in the beginning, and how very blessed I was now.

My thoughts went to other cancer patients who acted upon the opinion of the doctors who weren't willing to give them a chance. I thought of those cancer patients who went home and died because they were told to; to those patients who weren't aware there are other choices. My heart went out to them. On a personal level I was grateful though, as things seemed to be going pretty smoothly for me. At least that's the idea I had.

It must have been time for another shot, because I got one without asking for it. It was about this time when my contact person at Karmanos approached me. I'll not mention names here, except to say the person in question was only a physician's aide, and I don't think her question was something my oncologist sent her to ask. Whoever dreamed the issue up was irrelevant to me. That fact was that I was blindsided.

I was taking a chemo treatment, waiting for the bag of drugs to disappear into my veins, when the person walked up to me and suggested that they do a biopsy on my liver. Huh?

"Why", I asked? She said that they (meaning the doctors, I guess) didn't know if that was cancer in my liver or not. Huh?

Every PET and CT scan I'd ever had showed that the liver had a whopping big tumor in it. The tumor wasn't filled with swamp gas; it was filled with cancer. So, what was going on? It gave me the willies. A whole litany of reasons for my objections came screaming to mind. The reaction I settled on was, "No".

If they wanted to do something with my liver, then what about radiation? Gees, I was already on enough chemo to float a good-sized boat. To the question of radiation, she said, "No". I asked why. She said, "Umm, it...well...it wouldn't work. Okay, I thought, nothing doing!

What was going on? I didn't know for sure, but I had the feeling I was about to become a specimen. You know...like a live cadaver. All I could think of, other than NO, was that when doctors believe you're going to die...they take it way too seriously. That's just one of many issues that we all have to question. Stay on your toes folks; you could get blindsided in a hurry. Truly, it frightened me.

## Oxaliplatin: Nerve damage

When my treatments began I was told that one of the chemo drugs could cause more problems than the others. The Oxaliplatin could cause my feet and hands to go numb due to nerve damage. But, when I got to the point where I couldn't button my blouse, they would cut back on that drug. However, things seemed to be going well so far, and they didn't want to cut back on the drug until they had to. So, I agreed.

By this time, I was about mid-way through the six-months of treatments. I had lost very little hair. The nausea I felt wasn't worth talking about, and occurred only slightly after the 5FU treatment was over. Then there were two days where I wanted to sleep more than usual, and when I wasn't all that hungry, but I could still eat. Other than that, I didn't appear to have cancer at all. If fact, there were a lot of people who didn't take my cancer seriously because I felt so good, and appeared to be healthy. Strangers weren't aware of my cancer at all. I had lost only fifteen pounds, but that was from the very beginning. Ten pounds of that, I'm guessing, was due to the depression over losing my husband and getting no help for nearly four months with the cancer. But, that was then, and this was now. I felt like I was winning. That's quite a testament to the Protocel®, the doctors, and well...that's quite a testament to it all.

There were no real surprises or problems as July approached. I hadn't been in a hospital in weeks, and I felt physically fit. I wasn't itching to run a marathon or pump iron, but I felt good. I had never felt a great deal of pain except for the acid reflux. And, by now, there was very little of that to deal with. My balance was way off, and remains dubious to this day. I do things like cut a corner to close and bump into doorjambs, or sometimes trip over my own feet. I guess I can blame that on the cancer treatments...can't I?

By now, I was beginning to feel the numbness in my feet and hands that I was warned about. I could still button my blouse, so the Oxaliplatin continued as always. Oh how I wish I had stopped taking that chemotherapy drug right then and there. It's been a full year since my last chemotherapy treatment and my hands and feet are still numb and very tender. But, I didn't ask them to stop the Oxaliplatin. Live and learn, I guess.

I had begun to count down to the last of my chemo treatments. I had three more to go. Three more trips...three more treatments. The treatments would soon be over. Yes! I had made it that far, and I knew the rest of the treatments would come and go just as everything else in life does. Oh, how I wanted the treatments to come to an end.

I had another CT scan late in July, which showed some tumors unchanged, while others were continuing to shrink. It didn't seem likely that the tumors would be gone by the end of my treatments. And, although the cancer cells were reduced in number, all the cancer sites were still there. Additionally, I had no way of knowing whether the cancer in my leg bone had grown or not because I hadn't had a bone scan since Detroit took over my care. But, I still had my Protocel®. I remembered the beginning again. How many ways are there to say how grateful a person can be?

## Gail

My cousin, Gail, had found out about my cancer through my mother. I hadn't seen Gail in years, but as soon as she got the news she came from Pennsylvania and spent nine days with me. She had a lot of information to offer, as her husband, Joe, was the one who was battling stage-4 lung cancer. His prognosis was sure death within four months unless he took chemotherapy treatments. He had part of his lung removed at Sloan Kettering Hospital in New York several months before our conversation. Shortly after his surgery he was getting ready for his first chemo treatment when he was told about Protocel®. He opted out of chemo to take only the Protocel®. All of that took place nearly a full year before I discussed it with Gail. Joe is doing very well and has been back to work for months. He is alive, and his cancer growth has stopped. He has cheated death for well over a year, and he's still going strong. He has never had a drop of chemotherapy or a single zap of radiation. Everyone does things a little differently, that's the way he chose to treat his cancer, and that's the way it has to be.

While they were at New York's Sloan Kettering Hospital they stayed at The Miracle House. The Miracle House is an organization that provides an inexpensive place for patients to stay while undergoing various types of treatments for their illnesses. You and your caregiver rent one of three bedrooms, while sharing the bathroom, living room and kitchen of an apartment with other patients. They're nice apartments in a safe neighborhood, and are rented for $40.00 a day. Typical rental costs in that area of New York, and for the size of these apartments, are in the neighborhood of four to six <u>thousand</u> dollars per month (I find that amount difficult to tell about and still breathe). Living in New York is a lot of things to a lot of people, but one thing it isn't…it isn't cheap. Traveling to and from treatments is accomplished by using the Port Authority bus system. Or, you can take taxicabs if you can afford it. They couldn't afford that. Tips are expected in New York on everything. It can get pretty expensive.

While Gail and Joe were there they were told about a different type of radiation, referred to as Radiowave Surgery. It's a treatment that a doctor at Cabrini Hospital in New York offers. Basically, the way this radiowave therapy works is that they shoot the radiowaves into a tumor at three different angles. The radiowave is limited only to the tumor, saving the rest of the body from any damaging effects. It was a rela-

123

tively new process, and one that seemed to work well. Gail looked into it for Joe, but because of the number of tumors on his lungs he wasn't a candidate, as the treatments would have done more harm than good.

I became interested in it after our talk. I wanted to rid my body of cancer just as quickly as I could. So I e-mailed the doctor there to see if I could be considered a candidate. I was, he said, and he asked for my medical records. I gathered together all the information I had and sent it to him. An appointment date was set for September 7th, which was shortly after my last chemotherapy treatment. Gail agreed to be my caregiver while in New York, which is a requirement. She and I became involved in planning our trip to New York.

Gail's nine-day visit came to an end, and it was time to get her to the airport for her return trip. I've got it covered. Right…

I left home in plenty of time to make the 90-minute trip. Right…

We missed the boarding window by five lousy minutes! After 9-11 when the time for boarding is up…it's up. The computers for that particular flight are shut down, and I was left standing holding her bag. So, we went to plan 'B'. We headed back home.

I was driving on 28th street in Grand Rapids and Gail was on the phone with her family trying to make excuses for me for allowing her to miss her flight. Then, out of the clear blue, Gail let out a yelp! Every hair on the back of my neck stood straight out.

"What!" I asked (yelled).

"There's a Salvation Army Store!" She answered.

"A what?"

"Pull in…right here! Pull in there."

Glad that I wouldn't be facing manslaughter charges for running over pedestrians, I pulled in and we went shopping. She found a 'Jones of New York' suit for me that fit like a glove. Must be that Jones of New York was something to nearly flat-line over, because she almost did. Okay, that was fun! In between chuckles over the whole situation, I wondered how I could have miscalculated the boarding window by five lousy minutes. However, I redeemed myself somewhat by getting her to her flight the next afternoon a full 30 minutes early. I knew I could do it. I just needed a little practice.

## The End of the Chemotherapy Treatments

I finished my chemo treatments on August 22, 2006. My doctor wanted to start me on a second round of chemo. I wasn't into that as I had come to think of the chemo drugs as a source of death and decomposer. I told him about the Radiowave surgery that I had interest in. He didn't appear to be familiar with that process. That was likely, I thought because he dealt only with chemotherapy. But, he didn't seem to have a problem with my interest in it. I agreed to come back for more chemotherapy if that became necessary. I knew, though, that even if the cancer came back with its old vengeance I wouldn't be taking more chemotherapy. I'd been given 612 hours of three chemotherapy drugs along with a drug booster in the course of six months. If that much chemotherapy hadn't killed all of the cancer, I felt sure that another 612 hours wouldn't either. The only thing more chemotherapy would do, as far as I could see, was do devastating damage to my already beat up body. I knew what the chemo drugs were capable of doing now, and I had come to fear them as much, or more, than the cancer itself. This time, though, my fear was backed up by fact. Chemotherapy involves literally poisoning the rapidly-growing cancer cells while also poisoning and destroying rapidly-growing healthy cells in all of the body's necessary equipment like the bone marrow, gastro-intestinal tract etc, and can cause organ damage, like liver, kidneys, heart, lungs, etc. I just felt as though my body had taken all the chemotherapy that it could reasonably take.

No more. Chemotherapy did all the good it could do, and all the bad I would allow. I was convinced that more chemotherapy would cause the sort of physical damage that may leave me dependent upon others for my personal care, and I decided to avoid that at all costs. I had to look at other options, and the Radiowave surgery looked like my next best bet. I felt I had little to loose and hopefully a great deal to gain. So far things were going pretty well, and I wanted to keep it that way. I had come a very long way. Make no mistake though; I was glad for the chance to be able to take the any kind of treatment that would help save my life. But, right from the horse's mouth, chemotherapy is extremely hard to get through.

As I left the treatment center a thought struck me. Let's see...according to the surgeon in Northern Michigan, shouldn't I have been dead by now? Humm... I think my date with the undertaker was scheduled for April... and here it is August. I believe I'm still alive. It appears that he was WRONG!

# New York

Gail made arrangements with the Miracle House for our stay, and it was decided we would take the Amtrak to New York so we didn't have to drive while in New York, (an extremely good idea). We would disembark in Grand Central Station where we would grab a cab to the Miracle House. As plans tend to go…this seemed like a good one.

Gail and I boarded the Amtrak train in Altoona Pennsylvania, stowed our luggage… with help, and settled in for a nice calm ride to New York. That part of our plan worked like a well-oiled machine. You just sort of sit there and watch some pretty amazing scenery fly by while thinking good thoughts. I did wonder how we would manage 'all that luggage' once we were in New York though. Oh well, let's not borrow trouble. Our train would take us where we needed to go, we would grab something on wheels, load our luggage, find a cab, and be off to the Miracle House. With that all settled in my mind I decided to take a nap. I would need it.

We arrived at Grand Central Station right on schedule. Then, we disembarked.

First impression? There were enough people in that building to start their own country, and everyone of them were in a hurry to get to...God knows where. Everyone, but us, knew precisely where they were, they knew where to get the carts with the wheels to transport their luggage, and most importantly, it appeared that they knew where the door was. Two thoughts came to mind while one foot was on the floor, and the other was still on the train. I wanted to know where the door was too, and I wondered if radiation, in New York, was all the important to me. Okay...it was. Then I noticed that, inasmuch as they were all in a frenzy trying to get where they thought they needed to be, they appeared to be bored. I wasn't bored.

Close you eyes. Now, think of something you would like to see. Keep your eyes closed...Now, think of things you might not like to see. Okay, open your eyes. You're in New York!

Have you ever been to New York? Photos that I'd seen just didn't relate anymore. There are no sufficient words to describe my impression of New York City the moment we pushed our way out of Grand Central Station and onto the street. I felt as though I'd been living on the moon until then. Good grief! I had been on a New York street for approximately five seconds, and all I wanted to do was beat a path for home. I felt a new and instantaneous understanding of culture shock. I defined it in completely different terms; terms that directly related to my immediate situation, and it didn't take long to do it. I guess you could call it a revelation, and you'd be close. You know how some people like to relate masses of people in a huge city, like New York, as resembling a parade of ants? I didn't.

I think Gail must have been looking for a cab...or something. I was just looking! We hailed a cab at Grand Central Station and asked the cabbie to take us to the Miracle house. He did just that, as he knew exactly where that was. Thank

God! Personally, I was thinking we were pretty clever for having gotten as far as we had. And that's what I get for thinking.

Our destination ended up being the Miracle House's headquarters that was smack dab in the center of downtown Manhattan, and had nothing to do with bathrooms and bedrooms, which by now we were both in need of. When I tell you we found ourselves plunked on a street corner sitting on our luggage in the midst of the tallest buildings, the brightest lights, the largest mass of humanity I'd ever been a witness to, the loudest drivers, the yellowiest mass of cabs, and an unimaginable display of confusion wasn't up for discussion. If there was anything funny about this, it was that they didn't seem to think what they were doing, where they were, or what was going on was the least bit unusual.

Well, I supposed that it wasn't all those things for *them,* but I can assure you...it was for me.

I had no clue what to do. Riding in a cab hadn't seemed to work, so I called the doctor's office and told them, as close as I could, where we were. I don't remember exactly the tone I used, but remember that they took me seriously. The lady at the doctor's office gave me the correct address, and Gail hailed another cab. We were on our way again.

If I was going to have a panic attack, right then would have been the perfect time and place for that sort of thing. Actually, I didn't seem to have the time for a panic attack. Besides, I didn't want to miss anything. I tried to keep my eyes open and my 'poise' in check.

We were now in the second taxi playing automobile-dodge-ball with other taxies. Gale was livid with the first cabby for dumping us in front of a building that we had no business being in front of. So, she had her own thoughts to occupy her mind. Humm... as I think about it now...New York didn't seem to frazzle Gail. Everyone has his or her own 'frazzle point', but evidently Gail's needed some other situation to trigger hers. I couldn't guess what that might be. If being in a New York taxi on 42$^{nd}$ Street in broad daylight didn't do it, well then maybe she just didn't have one. I'm normal; I have a frazzle point, and it was offering new options to the situation on a second-to-second basis. I could have closed my eyes I guess; except that I didn't think that would be such a good idea. Okay, I thought, now that you know you are truly a roaring hick; what did you expect? Give yourself a minute, I thought, you'll get used to it. Then, I thought, why should I get used to it, I don't live here!

I argued with myself all the way to the apartment. I truly don't remember what I was chastising myself about. It didn't matter then, and it doesn't matter now. It kept my mind off the cabby's driving. I considered the chastising a form passive self-defense. You know; keep your mind off what could end up being the total destruction of your life as you knew it. It worked fairly well. Well...it worked.

Being from Mid-Michigan in a small town where the one traffic light blinks only yellow after the sun goes down, I found New York's traffic to be a curious thing. Okay, maybe not curious...maybe getting from one end of the block to the other end of the block in a car was a wonder of unspeakable magnitude. I wouldn't attempt to drive my car there for any reason that I could think of. I'm just not that brave, and I knew I surely had no talent for it. I would have had traffic backed up all the way to the Pennsylvania border in no time at all. Then there was the reality that someone would have clearly put me out of my misery before I got too far, and that could very well have been from a fireman's wrath.

You wouldn't believe how difficult it is to get a full-size fire truck around a corner, let alone to a fire, in Manhattan. I've seen firemen have to 'literally' get out of their stranded truck and direct traffic so they could find a sliver of space in order to be on their way. If you want a lesson in how it feels to look really dim-witted, get yourself stuck in Manhattan traffic with a full-sized fire truck behind you with its siren screaming like a mashed cat, and you have no place to go. That would do it for me.

What a fire truck needs in an emergency is an open road. The only thing that would open a road in Manhattan would be a lightening bolt from God himself. Then, all that would have accomplished would have been a full-blown panic. It would compound the fiasco and leave open the only other reasonable option, and that would be to merely get out of your car and walk away. Knowing what a nightmare traffic is on a daily basis, just think how it would be without their subway and bus systems. Hollywood couldn't come up with a bigger disaster.

There are so many sirens and horns blowing on New York streets that the drivers have become deaf to the noise, but they just keep on doing it. I know about the noise because Fire Station #1 was less than a block from our apartment. That would also put Fire Station #1 less than a block from our bedroom window. I'll bet that, in Manhattan, sleeping pills are the drug of choice. But, I digress. I'm getting ahead of myself.

We arrived at the apartment building, got out of the cab, unloaded our luggage and went straight to the apartment. That's where our very own bathroom was. I don't remember which of us was gracious enough to let the other go first, but whom ever it was deserves recognition of the highest form. Likely it wasn't me, as I had had all of the emotional trauma that my bladder could handle.

I thought about sleep for a moment. When nighttime comes in New York City you think of sleep just like you would if you were home. When you think of sleep, you think of quiet no matter where you are. Neither sleep, and surely not quiet, truly applies in New York City. Then, add the fact that there is no such thing as dark. I was betting that sleep would be a bit illusive at best.

Noise is the big problem though. New Yorkers drive with one hand on their steering wheel and the other on their horn. The streets are loaded and noisy, and that's an all day/all night thing. Blowing horns in Manhattan has a different meaning there than it does where I come from. They're in the midst of the greatest mass of cars, trucks, busses, fire equipment, police, and pedestrians that I've ever been a witness to...even in dreams. Blowing horns in New York isn't so much a plea to get out of the way as it is a vent for an emotional volcano eruption. It's a bad situation as far as I could see, and not something I wanted any involvement in. Just know that noise carries just as well in New York City as it does anywhere else... maybe better.

## Our first day ...

Confusion, noise, and dumfounded sights were compounded as we found ourselves in the middle of Manhattan while the United Nations was in session. That's a whole other story folks.

When the United Nations is in session, two of the main thoroughfares are closed down for the duration. Can you imagine how the fire and police departments look forward to the United Nations being in session? Not to mention the Port Authority's bus system. If traffic was a problem before, it was a mass of complete stupefaction then. I know...it unfolded before my very eyes.

There were motorcycle police at the cross streets clearing traffic for the parade of dignitaries that would soon pass by at a very high rate of speed. (And here I want to suggest that you really need to pay attention to the police, as they didn't appear to be kidding). Then came the black SUV's with tinted windows and, I'm betting, with gun packing CIA agents hidden inside. Behind them were the stretch limos, and then, came more black SUV's. Okay, I'll bet you've watched scenes like this on television. I have. But, let me tell you...seeing it as it unfolds in real time gave me a whole new perspective.

It almost made me feel as though I should be throwing myself over the hood of the nearest car just to get the formalities out of the way before they came to arrest me for... well...looking funny. And, here's another thing. If you think you have a good reason for carrying a concealed weapon at that moment in New York's history, I would suggest that you find the nearest storm drain and give it a pitch. Your day will become less *mixed up* if you choose to do that. I will tell you that we were awe struck with the sight, and you can believe it to be true. Likely, we were the only two women watching with slackened jaws. Of course, after the procession passed, the horn blowing resumed once again. What...a...city!

## Back to the battle

My consultation with the doctor went well. He's a funny and compassionate doctor. There was no intimidation, whatsoever, during my visit with him. He explained the procedure so I could understand, he ordered all the appropriate tests, and set a date for the formation of my Kayak (Kayak: my definition).

The tests came first. I was given another CT scan and another bone-scan. The CT scan determined that the tumors in my liver, colon, and the one on my aorta were the ones that the radiowave therapy would target, as they were the ones that were likely to kill me first. Yet another happy thought. The bone scan showed that the cancer in my left leg was completely gone. Another true testament for Protocel® as chemotherapy would have never even touched the cancer in the bone of my leg, according to my doctor at Karmanos in Detroit. I had to think what could have happened to me if just the cancer in my bone had begun to rip through me, not to mention the rest of the cancer sites. Not a happy thought at all. But, as you can see, that wasn't something I had to worry about anymore.

Then came the fitting for the Kayak, which is a body form that is used to assure your body doesn't move at all during the radiowave treatments. I was taken into a room void of heat, but there's a good reason for the coolness... I guess. I was given another huge hospital gown to wear, instructed to lie on the examination table over a black plastic bag, and there was a technician on either side of the table. One of the technicians began pouring some sort of liquid into the plastic bag. Soon, the liquid began growing and filling the bag, which formed around me and warmed my chilly body. I lay there giving the forming liquid time to set while enjoying the warmth it offered. The whole procedure took less than 45 minutes. With my Kayak at the ready, it was time for more instructions from the doctor.

Gail and I went in to see the doctor once more. He gave me a list of appointment dates, told me not to worry, and to enjoy New York while I was there. To his credit, he never mentioned death once. Well, that's not entirely true. While in a conversation with him on the phone before I went to New York, he agreed with the other doctors that I was terminal and the cancer would take my life...no matter what. I suggested that further treatments were of little use then. He reminded me that I could be 'run over by a truck' too. So far, that's about as much sense as any of them had made about my prognosis, so I decided to go on with it. I would never know if the radiowave surgery would work for me unless I tried, and it beat being run over by a truck. I hadn't thought that would be likely, but that's before I got to New York.

I would have my first radiation treatment the beginning of the following week. We left his office and took the bus back to our apartment. I have to say that I was excited about seeing New York. I didn't think I would ever get another chance to return, and I wanted to make the best of the opportunity I had to explore. We got some sleep, and readied ourselves for the weekend.

## We hit the streets

God loves Gail, and big business loves all women who live to shop. We were in New York City where there are more places to shop than any other place on the face of this good earth. We didn't hit them all, but we made an impressive dent. Thinking about it now, I guess I don't think there is anything you can't buy in New York. Some things are more difficult to find then others though. American food is one of those things. If you aren't into ethnic eating; pack a lunch.

By now my feet and hands were numb from the chemotherapy treatments (and, no, I couldn't button my blouse anymore). That made walking a test of endurance, but doable. After all, we were going to see as much of New York as we could, and I needed my feet to do that. Gail has a bum knee, but that didn't stop her either. If reality doesn't come between a woman and her shopping, then it's not too much of a leap to suggest that ailing feet and knees would either.

On the morning of September 11th we went to Ground Zero. I don't have much say about that except to say that you can't see something like that without being moved to tears. Seeing it in person makes it personal to you. It isn't a picture on television any more, or stories in the newspaper. It was real: it happened. It's difficult to imagine the carnage caused that day. People, just like us, were murdered in such a horrific way that it's impossible to fathom. Ground Zero is a massive hole in the fabric of humanity that opened up the hearts of the world. I believe that to be true for several reasons, mostly, it seemed that most of the rest of the world was there.

We had heard about the 'Ground Zero Light Beam', and so were anxious to see it that evening. Our apartment building had 44 floors (short by New York's standards), so we figured that the rooftop would be a good place to go to see it. On the evening of September 11<sup>th</sup> we went to the rooftop to take a look. The sight of the New York lights at night along with the spectacle of the light beam took my breath away. I will *never* forget that sight! Like little kids, we trotted from one side of the rooftop to the other to view the magnificent sight. If you've never seen it... you should. However, take a camera that works. I'd forgotten mine, and Gail's had a dead battery in hers. A picture would have been great to show our friends, but the picture your mind's-eye implants is there forever.

The following day would be the beginning of my radio-wave treatments, so we headed to the apartment to take a stab at sleeping again. In the morning we would become involved in Manhattan's mass transit bus system. At the very least, I thought, we were in for some mind-blowing confusion. You have no idea how right I was.

It came time to catch our bus for my first treatment. Now is as good a time as any to introduce 'Chemo-Brain'. Chemo-Brain is a condition caused from taking chemotherapy, and does some sort of damage to your memory. Whether it was long-term or short-term memory loss really wasn't the issue. It's a loss of memory. It's always better to have all of your wits about you while in New York. I didn't.

I could have gotten to the bus stop by myself, but that's where my prowess ended. Gail would look at me and say, "No, this way", or "that way." I watched her like a hawk to see which way she turned when we got off the bus. She had to think I'd lost my sense of direction or was just plain stupid, because she had to drag me all over New York City.

I truly hated that because I am an independent person, and found myself in a very dependent situation.

Being led around by an emotional tether was very degrading. However, the next time we left the apartment for a treatment she had to drag me all over again. I just couldn't find my bearings. It's a very good thing that she was with me. If she hadn't been, I doubt that I would have had to worry about the effects of the treatments, as I would have never found the hospital in order for the treatments to begin. That's how bad it was. I'll plead now what I pled then...Chemo-Brain. See how that works? She got me to the hospital, and I got through my first treatment without a hitch.

Right from the first day, the technician that took me to the treatment room referred to me as a 'Dear Lady'. Anyone who refers to me as a dear lady will be forgiven almost anything. When I got to the treatment room, I crawled into my Kayak, and was measured in a dozen different ways. Then, the lights went down, and the hum of the radiowave machine lulled me to sleep. As far as I know, it's the only place in New York where car and taxi horns go unheard. Cozy.

When my treatment was over I would find Gail waiting patiently in the lobby. She is my blood cousin, so I know that patience isn't her strong suite. But, she never complained once. Here she was away from her family, in New York, happily being a caregiver to a cousin she hadn't seen in years. That is the love for others that the Bible talks about, and a lesson for me to remember. It's the sort of love that says, "I'm filling your need just because I care".

## Seeing the Sights

We went to Madam Truedo's House of Wax during our first week in New York. Whoppie Goldberg's figure was standing by a post when we entered the museum. My first reaction was to step out of her way. My second thought was to 'get a grip'. Most of the presidents were there. For the most part, I'm not a political person as I view politics as a huge machine that has very little to do with the welfare of the little man (or woman), and a machine that is best avoided until voting day. But, there was one president there that I would have wrapped up along side his head had he been 'in the flesh'. The others, though, were just men made of wax... like always. There were some rock bands from my ancient past that I was mesmerized by, and of course, Superman was there in all of his glory. He made me think that perfecting his mode of travel would be a handy thing to learn to do in Manhattan. Most of the figures there brought back some sort of memory; some good...some bad. All in all it was one of many pleasant 'other world' experiences that the city of New York has to offer. I'm glad that we had a chance to see it.

Leaving the museum brought us out into the street again where reality resumed with all the noise, people, cars, and busses. I was beginning to get somewhat used to it.

The following week we took a boat tour, which included a close-up view of the Statue of Liberty. Any difficulty I've had with the way politicians run our country became second to the sight of her; but only until the moment passed. I was totally impressed with the size of her, and felt the pride I'd guess others have felt when seeing her for the first time. She is absolutely huge, she is totally remarkable, and she doesn't look at all French.

In general, other places and things, like Wall Street, look totally different than I thought they would. I can't really define what I mean by that the way I would like to, except to say that pictures aren't the real deal...not even close. The whole city is something you would have to see in person in order to get a feel for it. Being the country girl that I am, I wouldn't live in New York, but I would go back and spend a few days when I felt the need to be truly wowed. Also, I would have a hand-held GPS with me to help navigate the jungle. If you need to do something to spice up your life... New York is the place to get it done. It's also a very good place to go for excellent medical treatment.

I met patients in New York that made my battle with cancer seem easier somehow. There were two patients who had very little hope, as their cancer was caused from asbestos poisoning. Then, there was Mary. She was a 76-year-old lady who had fought her cancer for ten years, and was loosing the battle. Mary was a lady who you loved... just because. There was the lady who had been at the Miracle House for nearly a full year taking treatments and battling colon cancer as well. Also, a young man who was too weak to leave his room except for treatments, and a dozen more who were in dire conditions from cancer and other illnesses. God bless them all.

There is an interesting story about the 76-year-old Mary. Even in all of her pain and suffering, being wheelchair bound, and in her later years; she was a real comic. She would say some of the funniest things, and usually they were totally off the wall. While at one of her last treatments, however, she asked her doctor how much time she had left. She was told that she had less than three months left to live. That's quite a blow when your hopes for the survival of someone you care about is so intense. Gail and I felt pretty bad about the news. Mary's daughter was devastated.

Her daughter asked me about 'that stuff' I was taking (the Protocel®, everyone calls it 'stuff'), and so I explained all about it again. She wanted her mom to begin taking it. Time was an issue, so Gail and I offered to give her some of mine until they could get their own ordered. Because Protocel® works very well with radiation I felt encouraged, but hoped her body hadn't sustained so much damage from the conventional treatments and the cancer itself that even Protocel® couldn't help. She was willing to give it a try, so we set her up with the formula 50, and with the same dosage that I was taking.

There was a way of life that Mary and her daughter, Susan, had worked out. Mary would call Susan from her bedroom; Susan would scurry in to help her mom out of bed so she could use the bathroom. They would wrap each other's arms around the other's neck; Susan would pull Mary into a sitting position, and then lift her legs over the side of the bed. Mary would slip into a standing position. Susan would walk backwards while holding onto her mom, and the two of them would shuffle into the bathroom. When Mary was finished, the process was repeated in reverse.

Then, just four days after Mary began taking the Protocel® she called Susan from the bedroom. This time, when Susan went to her mom's room, Mary was out of bed and standing by the bedroom door. She had felt strong enough to get out of bed on her own. Getting settled in the bathroom would still require her daughter's help. I found it pretty amazing that she even get out of bed by herself, though and I was greatly encouraged. She even got some of her appetite back, and it was easier for her to swallow her food. Sadly though, the day I returned home, I received a call and was told Mary had passed away. The cancer and all the traditional treatments had just been too much for her frail body to handle. But, for those few days she was stronger. If Mary had known about Protocel® even a year earlier, I believe that she could very well be still alive today. It's my understanding that Protocel® has been available since the 1950's. I wish she had known.

My radiowave treatments went well for me. I kept taking my Protocel® throughout the all of the treatments, so the only difficulty I felt was a very slight case of nausea once in a while, which depended entirely on which particular tumor was being zapped that day. So, being in New York during that time was more of a vacation than a time for more treatments, as I rarely felt nauseated. Other than the condition that my feet and fingers were in, I felt pretty good.

The eleven treatments went without a hitch and they came to an end. During my last visit with my doctor, he asked that a CT scan be taken in three months. It could take that long, he said, to see how fast the radiowave treatments were working. He gave me a big hug, and Gail and I were on our way. Joe would drive into New York, pick us up, and take us home. That was another milestone behind me. Yahoo!

As I left the city, I knew that New York was the most amazing place I could have ever have imagined. But, being from a quieter and less congested world, I was glad to be going home. I can't imagine what sights and sounds real 'globe trotters' have tucked away in their memories. I'll bet their stories would be interesting to hear though.

# Back to Michigan

I had intended to stay with Gail and Joe for another two or three days. However, I had been on the road and away from home for the better part of eight months. I was getting homesick. Once I found my way out of the back roads of Pennsylvania (remember the chemo brain), I was headed home for good. However, I was only two or three hours into my trip when depression began to settle in. Why now, I wondered. I knew I would miss Gail, but I knew that the treatments were behind me now. I should have been elated.

Then, reality tapped me on my shoulder. I knew I had to face Dale's death. I had just begun the grieving process when the cancer was found. From the day I was diagnosed until my trip home from Pennsylvania my world was filled with cancer. I had to find someone who would help me with it, and then, how to begin destroying it. I had been too busy to grieve much at all. All during my treatments, going to New York, and dealing with the cancer, most of the grieving for my husband was stalled. I thought I would rather take a beating than face the grieving process with its full force. I came though.

You can put off grieving if you need to, but not forever. I never knew when I would start crying again. Most of the time some little thing on television triggered it. Or, maybe I would run across his toothbrush or jacket. Memories that would appear from nowhere would bring it on.

My mind began replaying his death scene over and over again. I was tired of fighting, so I just let it play out.

Dale had what he thought was heartburn or acid reflux. I suggested he call and get an appointment to see our family physician. He called, and was told the receptionist would call back with an appointment date. However, when the return call came in he was told he didn't need to been seen, and that he should take OTC Prolosec to ease his discomfort. Trusting the doctor... he did as he was told. (I truly hate that part...where he did what he was told to do!)

He kept waiting for the Prolosec to work, but it didn't. His heartburn was acting differently from one day to the next. For instance, we went to a picnic one afternoon where he ate things like hot dogs that should have set his heartburn afire. But, it didn't seem to be an issue. Other days, he had eaten things that shouldn't have bothered him at all, but did. We were beginning to wonder what was truly going on. After two and a half weeks something should have changed. If it really was heartburn then the Prolosec should either have eased the pain or not have worked at all.

We decided to go fishing the Sunday morning following the picnic. But, as we were making our plans the phone rang. Kam was swamped at the restaurant and asked if we could give her a hand. Dale said he didn't mind helping her out, so we showered, dressed, and left for the restaurant.

His heartburn was bothering him that morning, but he didn't seem to be in all that much pain. He looked okay, but it didn't occur to me that I was looking at a very sick man. He was in a good mood, and if he was worried about anything he didn't say anything to me about it. One of the things that hurts so badly is that he was less than 15 minutes from his death, and I had no clue.

He parked the car. When we entered the restaurant, he took off for the dining area, and I headed for the kitchen. We had been there less than five minutes when I saw him walking up to me out of the corner of my eye. If I had only known.

I knew it was Dale, but I didn't make eye contact with him. I don't know if he knew what was happening, but he had to know that something was terribly wrong. He headed for the only person he felt could help him...me. I was too busy doing something completely useless to meet his eyes. I didn't connect with the person who had become the other half of my life when he needed me the most; when he would need me so very desperately. He had walked close enough to touch me, and then he collapsed. I heard him drop, and I felt the air part as he passed through it. There are no words...

I dropped to my knees beside him just as he released the last breath he would ever take. I heard something like a gurgle or a rattle, and the emptiness in his eyes frightened me. But, I couldn't entertain the idea that he was gone. I kept telling him he was going to be all right. Then I began begging him to hang on. Then I started yelling for help.

At first no one came, but a second seemed like an hour. Dale and I were in an airless empty pit. There was no sound, nothing inside or outside of the sphere we had been slammed into. *It just wasn't real.* Then, out of nowhere a man took hold of my shoulders and moved me away from Dale. He was a big man from a motorcycle club who had come to help us.

The man began working on Dale as we waited for the ambulance. We waited and we waited. All the time we waited the man never left Dale's side. He kept up the compressions. Ten minutes, fifteen minutes, a half hour, and the ambulance still hadn't arrived. The man kept up the compressions.

People were everywhere, and the man kept up the compressions. Then, finally, the volunteer EMS unit arrived.

Shawn, an EMT at the time, was the first to reach us. As Shawn passed by, he looked at me in confusion. What was I doing there? I looked at him and said, "Bring him back, Shawn". He didn't answer me as he headed for the man on the floor. He didn't know it was Dale.

Shawn and Dale had been like father and son for years, and when Shawn realized who he was working on he completely broke down. The rest of the unit moved Shawn out of the way and took over. The big man who had tried so hard to save Dale's life stood, looked at me with deeply saddened eyes, and he walked away. He had worked so hard.

Shawn found me. He was sobbing. He told me that it didn't look good, and he held me in his arms. There was nothing more Shawn and I could do. Angie, Shawn's wife, was crying. People were praying. Others were on phones trying to connect with anyone who could help. Everyone wanted to help in any way they could.

The EMS crew cut Dale's shirt away from him then hooked him to the defibrillator and began shocking him in between respiration and compression efforts. They continued shocking him as they loaded him into the ambulance. Shawn and Angie grabbed me and we headed for the hospital.

I got to the room in the hospital where they were working on Dale. His bed was completely surrounded by doctors and nurses. As I took Dale's hand in mine they pronounced him dead. The doctor stepped away from Dale with tears streaming from his eyes. I wasn't crying. Dale died of a massive heart attack. I don't remember much after that.

I don't even like to look at the doctor's professional building, as I get angry all over again. I think Dale could still be alive if the doctor would have just taken a look at him…if she had just done her job. How dammed long could that have taken! But, she didn't, and now Dale was gone. I could have sued her with a vengeful gusto, but decided against it. I don't know why, except that vengeance or her money and reputation wouldn't bring Dale back, and that's all I had really wanted. That was something that was too late for her to give. I wonder if she lives with that.

## Finding a GP

I wouldn't have thought that finding a family-type doctor would be a big deal. But, it would prove to be. I wasn't about to go back to the doctor that Dale and I had before he died. I needed help, and that wasn't her 'bag'.

I thought the doctor who did the biopsy that past November would be a good bet. He wasn't an oncologist, or a GP, but he had some of my history. So, I set up an appointment with him. I had three small tumor-like lumps across the mid-section of my body that would cause a little discomfort at times. I asked him if he would remove them and have them biopsied.

He wanted me to go all the way to back down to Detroit to see my oncologist before he did anything, but didn't explain why he thought that was necessary. He wasn't satisfied when I said I didn't see what good that would do. It was probable the oncologist would suggest more chemotherapy, as without having another CT scan so soon after the radiowave treatments; I had to assume that I still had cancer in all, or most of, the same places. I didn't want to take more chemotherapy, and told him that. He didn't appear to be happy with my decision, but finally, he agreed to do the surgery.

I wish he had explained why he felt it was so important for me to see my oncologist before he felt good about treating me. But, he didn't. I don't know if doctors expect us to use mental telepathy to grasp their logic for what they say or do, or if they think we're just too dense to comprehend their reasoning. Maybe they expect our blind trust in their decisions concerning our health care. It's very possible they think we don't really care what they do just as long as they give us the pill we need to pacify our discomfort. Who knows? A little explanation would have gone a long way though. It's a little like keeping them in the dark when they ask us why we needed to see them. The conversation could go something like this...

"You're the doctor. Why should I waste my time discussing my problem? I'm paying you a lot of money and I expect you to know why I'm here to see you!" "Besides, I'm late for my next appointment with the hairdresser (or something as profoundly mundane). Of course, that could be easily dismissed by the doctor because the topic of discussion has nothing to do with his discomfort. It sort of reminds me of waiting in line at Wal-Mart. NEXT!

Nothing about a lack of communications between a doctor and the patient, or anyone else for that matter, makes much sense to me at all.

A week or so after the decision was made the surgery was done. One of the tumors had attached itself to my ribcage, and was likely the cause of the discomfort I had been feeling. However, all of the tumors were found to be benign.

During the post-op visit, he suggested that I have a couple of tests to check to see how much damage the chemotherapy treatments had done to my esophagus. Also, it was time for the CT scan that New York wanted. The appointment was set for the scan, and the other tests would follow that. Things seemed to be going okay as far as I was concerned.

Then, out of the blue, I got a call from his receptionist a week or so after my post-op visit. I was told that he wouldn't treat me anymore, and that I should look for another doctor. The CT scan and both of the other tests had been cancelled. I couldn't believe what I was hearing. I asked her why. All she would say was that it was complicated. Here we go again, I thought.

"Complicated?" I asked. "How could a couple of tests and a CT scan be complicated?" She said I just didn't understand, but that I should just accept that the situation was complicated and find another doctor. I'm still not sure I understand what happened that could have been so bad that the doctor wouldn't treat me, but that was that. She didn't seem to want to give me an explanation; so maybe retaining this doctor wasn't such a good idea after all. Good idea or bad idea wasn't the issue. Once again, I wasn't given answers or choices, and so I wasn't given the privilege of an understanding for their reasoning.

Doctors who pull the rug out from under my feet, for reasons that I'm not privy to, give me pause to think. Shouldn't my doctor be the one who takes charge of the situation? If he is only willing to help those patients who aren't *all that sick*, or those who won't likely present a challenge; then, I don't see the overall value in them. I would like to think that my doctor isn't more frightened of cancer than I am. If he is only willing to go so far, and I have to take up the rest of the slack...shouldn't we split his fees? Wouldn't splitting his fees give *him* pause to think? I may have struck on a groundbreaking solution for the lack of good rural medical health care in corner of the world. However, while I'm thinking what a humorous thought that may be, I'll be out looking for another doctor, yet again.

In a past life I had worked in the administration office of our local hospital. I called one of the doctors I remembered and asked him for the name of a good family physician. This doctor wasn't in practice anymore, but he gave me the name of a doctor he would send his family to, which is quite a recommendation. I called and was given an appointment.

I was leery about telling this new GP about the cancer, as I thought he would be afraid to treat me, or would refer me to another oncologist. I was getting very weary of being the leper who had cancer, but didn't think pouting about it would solve a great deal. Besides, it wasn't like he wouldn't have found out sooner or later. You know...like...

"Hey Elaine, how come you have all of these little pinpoint tattoos all over you?" Or, "I see a lot of scars. Did you get caught in a lawnmower or something?"

In the end I told him about the cancer. He alluded to an oncologist at one point, and I told him I had a very capable oncologist who I could see if it became necessary. Then I told him how I felt about more chemotherapy, and how I wanted to remain independent. He understood completely, and said that all he wanted for me was what was best for me. I told him I thought that, right then, he was what was best for me. I assured him that if my cancer came back, and I died, I wouldn't hold it against him. Thank goodness he had a sense of humor, as he gave me a smile and agreed to treat me. I thought we would have a good patient/physician relationship that should bring good results. With that, he began to devise the proper plan to get my health care under way. Yes!

First, there had to be CEA-125 blood test, and another CT scan taken. I told him that I had an allergy to the red dye in the contrast, so he ordered one using another type of dye. Because a different type of contrast was used the results came back somewhat cloudy, but were still reasonably readable. The tumor in my liver showed up as it had in the New York scan five months earlier, but was now in a wedge-shape, which is pretty unusual. There was no sign of the tumor that was positioned by my aorta, and my kidneys appeared clear of cancer as well.

The tumor on the adrenal gland was still visible, but he didn't seem to think it was cancerous. The cancer in my lymph nodes was still there, but was described as 'insignificant'. Radiation doesn't target lymph nodes, and I hadn't had a chemo treatment in six months. There is no question, as far as I'm concerned, that the reduction of cancer in my lymph nodes was a direct result of taking Protocel®. All in all, I was getting good news. Nothing was said about the tumor in the colon though. It must have been hiding, because I found out in a later test that it was still very much there.

The doctor didn't think the liver tumor was cancerous because it had changed from round to a wedge shape. However, he isn't into guesswork, so he ordered an MRI of that area just to be certain the cancer was truly gone.

Well, now I was in a bit of a pickle. I know, without a doubt, that I have to have the MRI. I tried to think of a way around it, but couldn't. The last time I had an MRI, I was in and out of the MRI machine twice before it could be finished. Claustrophobia is difficult for people to understand unless they suffer from it. I talked my fear of the MRI over with the doctor, and he said he would order a Xanax for the day of the test. One Xanax?

"Don't you have anything stronger", I asked?

"Well", he said. "I can make you stupid".

"Stupid is good", I said.

And so it was done. I was given stronger drugs, glided into the MRI machine with my eyes covered with a sleep mask, and I couldn't have cared less. Drugs can be *such* a good thing.

The MRI results proved that the liver tumor was no longer cancerous. It appears that the tumor was empty and was folding in on itself. I have a mental picture of the Radiowave surgery bubbling away on the inside of the tumor while the Protocel® was disintegrating the tumor's roots. Dr. Bell had told me months earlier that Protocel® would some- times attack and kill the roots of a tumor before it attacked the cancer cells inside the tumor. If that happens, he said, the cancer cells would starve to death with their food supply gone. If that happened, the empty tumor could change shape, and would either dissolve, or could be surgically removed. Either way, my liver was now void of cancer. The cancer in my liver was G.O.N.E.!

# CEA-125

The results of my CEA-125 (cancer marker blood test) revealed it to be a bit a little over the 5-point mark. My doctor said that was a slightly elevated result, but he wasn't concerned about it due to my history. It's important to know that when taking Protocel® and the cancer is dissipating, the patience's cancer blood marker test may begin to elevate. Tanya Harter Pierce explains it best in her book, <u>*Out Smart You Cancer*</u>, when she says; don't interpret this as a sign that your cancer is growing. Most cancer marker tests are *general* Indicators of how much cancer is in a person's body because they measure certain things that go along with, or are released by, that particular type of cancer cell into the bloodstream. For other types of cancer, the marker tests will be measuring a type of protein released by the cancer cells, and so forth. I had no reason to worry about an elevated CEA.

On February 21$^{st}$ I was given the PET scan the doctor had ordered earlier. The results of a PET scan are read according to the cancers density levels as opposed to centimeters and/or millimeters the way tumors are read in a CT scan. My doctor read the results to me, which showed there was no cancer visible anywhere, except in my colon. The tumor was about the size of a golf ball, and was described as being 'metabolically active'. He felt that the elevation of the CEA was due to that. It was apparent that the CEA was higher than normal due to the cancer that was left in my colon.

I didn't have a physician's understanding of exactly what metabolically active meant. But, I guessed the condensed version would be that it was still alive and active. I didn't know if it meant it would grow to a dangerous level in a short period of time, or if it meant it was in its final death throws. We decided to have the tumor surgically removed. It felt good to have a doctor who felt my opinion about <u>my</u> health was important. Finally!

The cancer in my liver and lymph nodes were gone! I had always believed that those were the two cancer sites that led the doctors to the prognosis that sent me to the funeral home months earlier. I couldn't believe my good fortune! Just as much as the original diagnosis was difficult to deal with, so was the conclusion that the cancer had been obliterated except for that one tumor. It was exceptional news, but somehow, difficult to take in.

I had to wait until the doctor could decide which local surgeon would do the best job. I was still taking my Protocel®, so I wasn't too worried about time. This time I was happy to await the doctor's call, as it would mean the last of the cancer would soon be taken away. God knows how happy that made me, and how anxious I was to have it over with.

In the meanwhile I went home and took care of things that I had been unable to look after while I was in treatment. I had many chores on my very own 'Honey Do' list, and knew I would be busy taking care of them for a good long time. Now I knew what Dale must have felt when I thought his 'Honey Do' list was essential to our well-being. Poor guy. At another time in my life I would have dreaded the work ahead of me. After I got into the list, though, I found the work to be somewhat therapeutic. You know…busy hands for idle minds…and all of that stuff.

I was at home picking up and cleaning things in the house while in a wonder about my progress. I hadn't re-opened my business yet as I still had the surgery to deal with. And, by that time I had very little to do with my list of chores fulfilled... sort of anyway. It was very cold outside and I wasn't anxious to go outside for any reason. Then, the phone rang, and it was Randy.

"Hi mom", he said, "I'm thinking about doing something, but you have to be flexible".

I had to smile at that. Flexible? I told him that flexibility was definitely in the cards for whatever he had in mind. He said that because my birthday was in March, and his wife's and my granddaughter's were in May that he would like to take us all to the Bahamas on a cruise. I thumped the ear I had to the phone and asked him to repeat himself. He did. Before he was finished repeating himself I was dancing all over the kitchen floor with wild abandon.

All that had been on my mind for the past 17 months was fighting cancer. Looking ahead for much of anything, and especially looking forward to the fun side of life, hadn't become a routine approach to the rest of my life yet. Oh yes! I could definitely deal with the Bahamas! Who couldn't! I may have had chemo-brain, but I wasn't stupid. Of course I wanted to go!

He works for an airline, and so I would fly to his house, at no cost, on stand-by.

I arrived in Georgia five days before we were to begin our trip. Randy took us shopping for warm-weather clothes, and so his wife could buy a gown for the big dinner night that is a tradition on a cruise. As they were shopping I looked around and found a white dress that looked like something a young model would wear barefoot on a sandy beach in a place where you never thought you would be. It was pretty, and it fit perfectly, but thinking whom it was designed for, I put it back on the rack. I was way past thinking I needed something like that to wear. My son smiled at me, took the dress back off the rack, and put it on a mountain of new clothes that was destined for the trip. He bought the dress for me. Now, all I had to do was figure a way to look young in it. Yea...right...

The Royal Caribbean ship stood in the harbor looking bigger than I could have dreamed, and it was impressive. Thinking about the depth of water that we would be floating over, I thought big and impressive was good, and I tried hard not to think about the lifeboats hanging securely on the side of the ship (details like that get my attention). We boarded.

The ship was designed to pamper you while taking you to places you've only read about. Places that are warm and inviting. Places that offered new experiences, sights, and sounds. Exciting? Exciting! We were on our way.

We sailed all the first night, and in the morning we found ourselves at a little island called Coco Key. Many of the Spring-Breakers were snorkeling off shore, while the rest of us were wandering around looking at the sights and eating whenever and whatever we wanted. Randy and his family went for a walk on one of the nature trails, while I sat in a beach chair watching the college kids doing what they do best...having fun. They were loud, and sometimes obnoxious, but were a great amount of fun to watch. I thought how, if I were that young; I would have been obnoxious right along with them. Knowing what I know now...I may have been even more obnoxious. What a happy thought.

Just as soon as we were back aboard the ship we were underway again. We were bound for Nassau. That evening was the big-dinner night. So, we all dressed to the nines and left for the dining room. It was packed with some of the best-dressed people I've seen in one room...ever. We fit right in. Yahoo!

There we ate some of the best food I've ever had the pleasure to indulge in. I watched waiters carry as many as twenty-five dinners on a tray, on a moving ship, through a large crowd of other waiters, while never once dropping even a spoon. Unbelievable! There was singing going on, people laughing, and smiling faces everywhere. And, I didn't drop a morsel of food on my white dress.

We docked in Nassau the following morning. We left the ship and began to look for some good cigars that Randy wanted; Cubans I think. He couldn't find exactly what he wanted, but found some very big cigars anyway: not Cuban.

Then we found ourselves at a really huge flee-market type buying experience that Gail would have died for. I bought an island-type dress that I was happy with, but one I would likely be very lucky to I find a place to wear once I got home. But, who cares...right? We were having fun.

I spent a good part of the next day leaning at the ship's rail trying to find an adequate name for the color of the ocean's water. I couldn't come up with anything that would convey the absolute beauty of the water. The inside of the desk was covered white with salt, which was a stark contrast to the ocean. It was definitely a different world there than I was used to in Michigan. Anything covered with white in Michigan equals...snow.

There are entertaining things going on all over the ship all the time. So, if you are the sort who likes to stay put, you can remain on the ship during the whole trip and still have a good time. There are well over 1000 people on that ship whose sole purpose it is to make you feel at home and completely comfortable. They do their job well. We had a completely wonderful time.

I stayed with Randy and his family for another day when we returned. Then, I flew home again, and began the process necessary to get the surgery underway.

## The surgery

Upon my return home I found that the doctor had made an appointment for me with a local general surgeon. Exercising choice, I thought about the expertise of a general surgeon, and then the expertise of a colorectal specialist. The specialist was a 220-drive away, but colorectal surgery is all the doctor does. He won. I'd been through too much and I'd come too far to take a chance on the general surgeon. Moreover, I hadn't been dropped on my head since birth. My Southfield doctor would know more about my cancer, he knew me, and I felt that I would gain better results from his skill. With that settled in my mind I decided to call for an appointment.

I was given an appointment for the 20th of March 2007. "It's getting closer" I thought. I almost felt giddy. I literally relished the thought of the surgery. Well, maybe not the surgery, but surely the result it would have on my cancer. What a feeling! What a wonder! What a blessing!

It had been seventeen months from the original diagnosis, just one year and one week after my first chemotherapy treatment, and eleven months after my first dose of Protocel®. The day I was given the appointment to see the surgeon was one full year from the month that my funeral should have taken place. It had taken one full year of a test of endurance to have the ability to hear the alarm clock, learn a new appreciation for life, and to feel the sun on my face. It was worth all the fear, the sickness, the disappointments, and the mileage on my body to be where I was that day. Was it finally over? Not yet, but it could be close to being over. I would find out for sure just how close it was after the surgery was done. God in Heaven... I felt alive again!

I was asked to fax the latest CT and PET scans to the doctor before the appointment day arrived. I did that, and then I made arrangements to stay with Duane and Karla until I recovered from the surgery. I left for Detroit on March 19th.

By this time Duane was back to work, so Karla and I had to find the doctor's office on our own. We didn't have Duane's GPS, and neither of us had a clue how to get to the doctor's office. Detroit is a very big city. We left *very* early, and it was a good thing because we got ourselves lost almost immediately after crossing into the city's limits. At one point we found ourselves in an area of Detroit where locked doors, closed windows, and not too much chitchat was in order. We turned around...again, and headed back to the main road.

On the main road we found that, on one side, the cross street was called one thing, and on the other side the same cross street was called something else. It was the 'something else' that we needed. Tell my why the people who name streets do that. Why can't a street have the same name from one end of it to the other end of it? I can get lost easily enough without their help, thank you very much. We have enough to deal with…right?

We finally found the doctor's office and I ran, numb feet and all, to beat the appointment clock. Karla and I made the appointment just in time. I thought that, even though I knew where several gas stations were located in Southfield, and any number of turn-around driveways, I wondered if I could find my way back to the doctor's office for further appointments. It's not like we took the most direct route to get there. If you find being directionally challenged strange, or difficult to understand, it is likely you aren't a woman. I think I'll get myself a GPS for Christmas. I wonder if Santa has a sense of humor, or if he feels the depth of pity I feel for myself when I'm totally lost. I could only hope.

We were called to the examination room and waited there until my doctor came in. He talked a bit about the cancer, and suggested that I have the surgery sooner than later. I wasn't in a huge amount of danger, he said. But, waiting wasn't going to improve matters either. I agreed, and it was decided I would have the surgery just as soon as he could arrange a hospital date. Actually, I suggested that the surgery take place just as soon as he could get my sorry self in the hospital. It would be done.

I was flying. I felt like a weighed as much as a feather. I wanted to dance, I felt like crying, I felt like hugging strangers (almost), and I wanted to drop to my knees and thank God for loving me, for guiding me to the doctors in Detroit, for the Protocel, and for the very air that I breathed. Being alive is a very good thing, but *feeling* alive is what it's all about!

My surgeon would have preferred that my oncologist examine me one last time before he did the surgery, and he explained why. He wasn't sure how much damage the chemotherapy and radiowaves had done to the colon area, and didn't want any surprises when he opened me up. I tried not to dwell on that part of it...you know...the part where he would 'open me up'. I have a vivid imagination. If I can't see it in a mirror...I don't want to see it.

I asked him if it could be worked out another way, as my finances had taken a real beating in the last year and a half. The cost of an additional oncologist's office visit is a considerable sum of money, and I wanted to eliminate the expense if it was possible. He said he would call and see if my oncologist could satisfy his questions over the phone.

It got a little interesting here. When he called the oncologist's office, he was told that the doctor was in, would be with him in a moment, then he was promptly put on hold. He was on 'hold' long enough to muster his anger. He sputtered, like we all do, that he was a busy person just as the oncologist was. *Indignant* would be a good word to describe his disposition. In his defense, he doesn't put his patients on hold. We are told he is busy, and that he will return the call. He always does. He finally got through to my oncologist and was able to speak with him before I left Detroit that day. He said he was completely satisfied with the conversation. Good deal!

My surgery was scheduled for the following Tuesday morning. He cautioned me that there could be three different outcomes from surgery. All three scenarios depended upon any pre-surgical damage to the surgical area. The best-case scenario was simply the removal of the tumor and colon along with a small amount of intestine to err on the side of caution. The worst-case scenario would be that I would have to wear a colostomy for the rest of my life. He tried to explain how, or why, the worst-case scenario would become necessary, and he lost me shortly after he opened his mouth. If he had drawn me a picture I still wouldn't have understood about all the twists and turns that would have taken place in my plumbing. But, you know what? At least he tried, and his trying made me feel better about the whole thing. At least I knew that *he* knew what he was talking about. I had to believe that the best-case scenario would be what he would be dealing with anyway. I don't know why I thought that, but I did. So, who cares why?

The other issue was my liver. He knew what the PET scan had shown, but he wasn't ready to believe my liver was truly clean of cancer. He wanted to make sure what was 'going on in there', so that was to be a priority during surgery as well. Also, he was sure he would find cancer in the part of the intestine that he decided he would remove. Beyond that, he predicted that I would be in the hospital for five to seven days, and that the surgery would last approximately three hours.

He needed information from New York, and any test results that were available from the last six months. I would have any other tests that were needed after being admitted to the hospital. In the meanwhile, I would get the information he needed before the weekend arrived. I dared to believe that this surgery would bring the nightmare of cancer to a final close. Hope was like a vibration. The surgery just had to work. And, by God's hand...it would!

I've been wrong before, so while I waited for that day to arrive, I wore my knees out praying that I wouldn't have to have a colostomy, and that the doctor wouldn't find more cancer other than the colon tumor, and I prayed from my very soul.

## The big day

Karla, and my niece, Robin, were with me the day of surgery. I was all prepped and ready, and everything was right on schedule. A nurse came to me and prayed with me, then put something in my IV. That's the last thing I remember until late in the afternoon when I woke up and I was in my room.

When I got my wits about me I prayed that I wouldn't sneeze. My surgical area hurt like crazy, but when I coughed I found myself in the midst of a personal emergency. I was given a pillow and was told to hold it tightly to my surgical area…then I could cough if I needed to. In fact, I was encouraged to cough. I have been given advice before that I didn't think was going to work well for me. At that time coughing – for no good reason – fell into that category nicely. However, when I learned that, without coughing, pneumonia could set in if I didn't cough… I coughed. Rats! They should try to come up with a better plan.

## The News I Had Been Waiting For…

Read this part carefully my friend. This is the part of the story that I had waited for from the very beginning. This is my message for *you*. Here is your reason to collide with cancer instead of giving in to it. While you're reading this part of my story, you'll find it easy to understand why I believed that my life was now measured by the moments that took my breath away.

My doctor spoke with my family after the surgery was over. He told them that after 25 years of doing this type of surgery he had *never* seen anything like it. He just shook his head in amazement. He found my liver to be *completely* clear of cancer and *healthy*. The intestine he removed for caution's sake was, in his words, *as clean as a whistle*. The density of cancer inside the colon tumor was minimal compared to the tumor's size. In addition, the surgery time was reduced from three hours to an hour and a half. Does it get any better? Sweet...

You're right there with me, right? I'm here for *you* right this minute. Believe with me that my success story can be your success story as well. Believe with me while I believe in you.

The student doctors who were in surgery with my doctor were young, and they were amazed by the outcome. A group of them visited my room every day. I got the impression that they thought of me as a wonder woman of sorts, because they hadn't found what they were sure they would fine...lots more cancer. The point here is that, without the care and concern of my doctors in Detroit and New York, and especially the Protocel®, I'm sure they would have found exactly what they had been looking for.

My surgeon stepped a little closer to my hospital bed during one of his visits with me. He asked me who told me I had only two months to live. I told him it was my oncologist from Karmanos. He was an oncologist that my surgeon knew quite well. I got the impression that he was trying to figure this whole 'clean liver' thing out, and was having difficulty making sense of it all. He said he was going to call him. That's all he said about it, and when the visit was over he left. I don't know if he actually called my oncologist. I didn't ask, but I assume he did. I would have liked to have been a fly-on-the-wall during that conversation. Wouldn't you?

I'm no wonder woman; far from it. I'm nothing special. But, the doctors who helped me are, and surely Protocel® is. Thank God for Jim Sheridan's willingness to spend his live developing a non-toxic product that helped save my life, and certainly for bringing me back to health. He has to be in a very special place in Heaven, as I'm sure God is "well pleased" with this great man. Someday, when I see him in

Heaven, I intend to give him a long crushing hug. I wonder if a spirit body can be crushed with a hug...oh well, we'll see. Thank God I had taken the Protocel® along with the chemotherapy drugs. Protocel® doesn't destroy anything in your body except the anaerobic cells. And, the antioxidants in the Protocel® helped maintain my immune system, which I believe helped keep my organs healthy. All the chemotherapy drugs in the world won't kill enough cancer to cure it before the drugs kill you first. That's just the way it is.

## Density Versus Size

During my post-op appointment with my surgeon, I asked about the density of the cancer cells (PET scan) as opposed to the size of the tumor (CAT scan). I couldn't picture in my mind what measuring cancer by density 'looked like'. He explained what that meant in terms that he thought I might understand. Now, let me see if I can get this right...

The more the cancer grows, or accumulates in one spot, the bigger its house (tumor) becomes. But, what happens when the cancer mass is dying? Well, as the cancer dies away the tumor will be larger than the cancer used to need. In other words, there is more room in the house than the residence needs. So, in order to get an accurate measurement of how much cancer really does exist, it has to be measured in density via a PET scan. The PET scan will show how much room the cancer takes up inside the tumor. The density in my colon tumor took up less than one-half inch of the space in the golf ball sized tumor. That impressed me a great deal, and apparently, it impressed my surgeon even more.

I like being impressed like that, but knowing that the cancer was gone was a totally surreal conception. It was the same as being told to go home and die...only it was a complete and utter turn around. It was just as difficult to take in. It hadn't hit home yet.

I was sitting in my car in my brother's driveway when it hit me. I broke down and cried in disbelief and relief. It was a long, scary, tough road to travel. It was the longest and most difficult battle I've ever faced. And, it's a mêlée I pray I never have to be involved in again. However, as bad as it was, I would fight just as hard if I had to do it all over again. The day I lay down for the last time I won't have to wonder if I had done everything I could do to hold on to the gift of life.

So, after all this time, after all the prayers, the Protocel®, the drugs, radiation, travel, good times, bad times, friends, family, bad nerves, nerves of steel, and whatever else needs to be thrown in…tests show no cancer! No cancer was visible in my body…anywhere!

I've been asked if I would quit taking Protocel® now that the cancer was gone. My answer is always a resounding, "No". I've battled cancer twice now. That's all the proof I need to understand that my body can't fight cancer cells off on its own. Cancer is a living, breathing monster that tries to take everything away from you. It wants your health, your faith in God, and your hope in the future. It wants your joy and happiness, and it wants you to give up. But, you *can't* do that. So, I will very likely take Protocel® for the rest of my life and be very grateful that that is all I'll ever have to do to keep cancer in its place. If that's all I have to do to stay healthy…I consider it a cakewalk.

# Back Home at Last

I was back home, and the surgery was over. My surgeon said that I had to be very careful about lifting much of anything for six weeks so I didn't rupture the surgical area. I thought that maybe a rupture would present itself as a bulge of some sort. My family doctor impressed upon me the significance of a surgical rupture. A surgical rupture could mean that the whole surgical area could open up. My immediate thought was of Super Glue…just in case. I lifted nothing heavier than a teacup as I dutifully waited out the six weeks, and was careful after that time was up as well.

I wanted and needed to get the store ready to re-open, and I had a ton of things that needed to be sorted for a garage sale. I busied myself with the tasks at hand, and as long as I was busy I felt fine emotionally. I hired the help I needed to do some electrical work, and to get some repairs completed. I made good progress while not over taxing my strength. My 'can't lift anything' time was over, so I began restocking the store and giving it a spit-shine. On July 2, 2007 I opened the door for business once again. It had been a long time coming. I stood in the middle of the store while the recent past zoomed across my mind. I can't tell you how I felt, because words aren't adequate. Sometimes it's just better to be still and feel. It felt like a true miracle and an awesome wonder.

Things were going as expected. Most of my previous customers had found others to do their embroidery when I couldn't, so being truly busy in my business would take a while to achieve. But, I knew it would happen. Soon the business would take off in the near future, just like it did before. But, the best of my future is today; it isn't down the road.

My future today looks and feels different than my future did before, even when Dale was still with me. Before, it was a sort of 'hurry up and get things done' sort of future. Now, it's like a new and gentler world is out there. I can touch it any time I want to. I know where I've been, and it doesn't matter so much where I'm going. I'll get where I need to be when I need to be there. It's a simpler way to live, but I like it that way.

I think about the way things began, and how things are now. This whole bout with cancer has shown me eighteen months of emotions that I never imagined that I would ever have to deal with, eighteen months of life changing events that took me places I would never have guessed I would visit, and a totally different view of life in general. Eighteen months ago I had less than two months to live. I was told to go home and die. I planned my own funeral because I had no hope. I felt desperate, desolate, and totally broken back then. I have faced death; but I am alive and I am well! When I think of all that has happened in the past eighteen months…I sit here in awe.

In the beginning every doctor I'd seen, whether they were oncologists or GPs, the good ones and the bad ones; they all said the same thing. Even if my cancer was put into remission, it would come back, and ultimately, it would take my life. As bad as chemotherapy is it stopped the cancer's rage long enough to give the Protocel® time to take over. When Protocel® got a grip on my cancer it didn't let go. The radiowave treatments helped as well. If the cancer ever comes back I have no reason to believe that God, Protocel, and my will to live won't keep me safe. That will give me emotionally assurance while it keeps me physically sound. So, you see...I believe it really is over. Oh God...it's finally over!

## Fight the Good Fight

Don't be afraid to try different courses and procedures, but only with good advice and with caution. If you're leery of a non-toxic product like Protocel®...put your fears to rest. It worked for me. There's not much doubt that all non-toxic products, or natural supplements won't work as they promise. However, that doesn't mean that all natural supplements are hoaxes. Protocel® did exactly what I needed it to do; it helped give my life back to me. I'm living proof of that fact.

There are several non-toxic products that have the ability to kill cancer cells, and none of them are laden with poisonous drugs. But, for me...Protocel® worked the quickest and was easiest to take. All I'm asking you to do is dig for answers. Find a way. Ask questions; be aware of your options. *Cancer: Step Outside the Box*, a book by Ty Bollinger that has a ton of good advice about surviving cancer. Buy it and read it. Make plans to do something important next year. Then, find something that works for you so you can be there to make it happen.

Have faith in yourself and the worthy physicians. They aren't all bad, but choose one carefully. Develop a strong and personal relationship with God. That is very important. He will be there for you. Try not to fall into the trap of fear that says your hopes will be dashed. Instead, think of the waste if you didn't allow hope to reign, and then realized too late that hope was the one missing element in the mix that could have helped save your life. Where hope is concerned, you have nothing to loose and everything to gain. Humor helped give me control over my fears. It could work that way for you as well.

Above all, if you don't consider yourself a fighter…learn to fight for your life. Fight hard! You're worth the effort. You've earned the right to live; you have the right to fight. You don't know what's around the corner for you. It could be that one thing you've been waiting for all of your life. You have to be there to catch the dream.

Life isn't tied with a bow, but it's still a gift. All you have to do is open it. So what if you have to untie knots. Maybe there's more debris inside your box than you anticipated. But, so what? Keep digging. You'll finally get to bottom of it. You'll have your life back in the end. You'll go on a journey with the side of love that you've not had the pleasure to know before your cancer hit you. *Just, please, fight!*

## Where I'm at Today

I knew that when I returned from New York I wanted to live just as much as I ever did. But, I knew that I couldn't, and wouldn't, take more conventional treatments, even though I knew that I still had a lot of cancer to deal with. I'd seen enough, read enough, and lived through enough to know that more chemotherapy drugs were surely not the answer, at least not for me. So, the only other option I had to kill the rest of the cancer was God first, then Protocel® and my resolve to live. All the doctors expected me to die. Somehow…I didn't.

I tried to forget that I had cancer at all (not easy, but mostly doable). I ate something nutritious every day, but I didn't eat a lot (I never have been a big eater). I never missed a dose of Protocel®, and I continued to drink a lot of water. Because I felt really connected to God, I didn't spend much time worrying. Not about cancer, and not about money. I gave myself time to recover from the conventional treatments, and I relished the life I had stolen from death.

I wanted desperately to help cancer patients get through their ordeal if I could. I wanted, with all my heart, to support any effort they could muster to beat the life out of their disease. I just didn't know how to do that. Then, God showed me a way. A friend suggested that I write this book as a source of encouragement for other cancer patients who were down-and-out like I had been.

Do you think you could write a book…about anything? Neither did I. But, I decided to try. If you knew how I began this book you would wonder how I got this far with it. And, if you had been there in the beginning of it, you would have laughed out loud. When I wasn't mentally wadding up page after page, I was in a quandary as to why I thought I could write anything…let alone a book. But, I did as God showed me. And, you're reading it now. Surely, if my story began to be easy to write, it was because God made it easy. I pray with all my heart that you find something; anything that I went through that will help you literally collide with your cancer. It isn't that I *think* you can do it. It isn't that at all. It's that I *know* you can do it. All you have to do is… do it.

If someone broke into your home with the intent to do you bodily harm you would grab a gun, a ball bat, or something to protect yourself. You would beat the intruder off. You would do that because you aren't going to roll over and let that person have his or her way. Right? Your cancer is now that intruder. Cancer is the evil that intends to do your body, mind, and soul harm. It's within your power, within your right, and within your reach to fight it out of you.

As for me, right this minute going on in life alone isn't as bad as I thought it would be. I stay busy, I count my blessings, and I tell myself in one way or the other that I'm healthy and happy, and I'm happy that I'm healthy.

## My Last CT Scan...

I had the three-month CT scan in June that was to be taken three months after my surgery was over. I'm happy to say that it showed no new growth of cancer. No tumors, no cancer, and no threat. I still had the numbness in my feet and fingers, and will likely have that for the rest of my life. My hair was back to normal; my emotions were as normal as they could have been under the circumstances, and I felt good to still be alive.

I felt as though I had just stepped out of the door and onto solid ground after traveling on a fast-moving long black train. But my emotions were bounding around like popping corn. It wasn't much of a surprise when I found myself smack-dap in the middle of a bout with mild depression, and so I took it to the doctor. He prescribed an anti-depressant for me with instructions to stay on them for nine months to a year. I'd been through a lot, he said. Because of all the stress my chemicals had likely become unbalanced. I couldn't argue with that. However, I have to confess that I wasn't happy about taking anti-depressants. I had to, however, keep my emotions in check. So, I took one each morning for five days, but began to feel worse (he had warned me that could happen).

In the meanwhile, it had begun to crack my veneer why so many doctors don't get the warm fuzzes where I'm concerned. I'm very leery about taking prescription drugs. Have you seen the warnings for side effects on the drugs you see on television these days? Of course you have. So, I'm watching and listening just like you are. I'm thinking to myself...would I rather find a natural therapy: something that won't attack another part of my body while it tries to rid my body of the depression? Or, do I want to trade this ailment for another one that could be much worse. I wanted to find a more natural route if I could find one.

In the end, I tossed the anti-depressants, got out my Sony Walkman, jammed the earplugs in as far as they would go, turned up the tunes and went on with life. That worked for me. Thank God for Vince Gill.

# Something to ponder

You know what? I don't know if there is someone out there who can wage a battle with cancer all by them selves. Maybe there is, but I'm not one of those people. I needed to know that my life, my presents, that part of me that makes me up was important to someone. All the people who were involved in my treatment and recovery were the foundation, the very hope that I so desperately needed to keep the fight alive.

However, I couldn't depend totally on others to drag me through the mire. I had to stand as tall as I could while they helped me through. When I got to the point when I couldn't seem to muster the faith I needed using my own strength, they let me borrow theirs. It was a team effort. It was sort of like what scuba divers do when they buddy-breathe. I'm not here because I was strong; I'm here because 'we' were strong.

I'm grateful first to God, then Protocel and the doctors who stuck with me. I'm eternally grateful to my big brother, and my son, for my mom and Reg, and a host of friends. I'm grateful for all of those angels more than I can ever express. The care, consideration, and support I've received in those

28 months from all of these people boggle my mind and soul.

All of those people were the army of angels that God sent to help me. They knocked on my door. They called me on the phone. I had get-well cards and e-mail messages from people I hadn't seen in months or even years. No friend or family member gave me the impression that they felt I wouldn't make it. They prayed for me. They told me jokes; they shed a few tears in my behalf. They're the army who picked me up when I didn't think I could get up. They let me talk about dying, and they let me talk about living. See? That's what angels do.

I've been asked if I believe I will ever get cancer back for the third time. I can't answer that, but I truly doubt it. All I know about is today. I know I'm still here over three years after I should have died. They've been three good and productive years. I still have God's love, Protocel's help, and my will to live. I think as many positive thoughts as I can. I remember to be truly grateful for the things I have, for the life I've been given, and for the people who love me. I fill as much of my life with humor as I can, and I try to give aid and comfort to as many people as will allow it. That's all I know... That's good enough.

# The end of the battle

I've waited a while before I published this book for a good reason. I've had a lot to say about doctors, treatments, death, life, and a lot of other things. But, not much of that would have mattered to you unless you and I knew that the cancer was truly gone. I didn't believe that one doctor or one report was conclusive evidence of that. So, I waited one full year after my colorectal surgery, and eight months after my last CAT scan was taken.

I had a literal battery of test taken on everything I couldn't see in the mirror. They included a physical examination, a CEA125, other blood work, urinalysis, a mammogram, ultra sound, a chest x-ray, and a PET scan. Everything came back normal. No pathologic areas of hypermetabolic activity at all...anywhere. Nothing, zilch, zero. The cancer is gone. I'm no longer dying. I'm not in remission. Praise God in Heaven...I'm cancer free!

You'll notice that my CEA125 results were 5. My doctor told me that a reading of 21 is within the normal range. Anything over 21 could be an indication that the cancer *could* come back. It's now obvious to me that I may just die of old age...somewhere further down the line, and it won't be due to cancer! Moreover, my immune system is in very good shape. A good immune system indicated to her that my spinal fluid isn't contaminated with cancer either. I hadn't thought of that possibility, and am very glad I hadn't.

So there you have it: the final proof. Read my reports. Know that cancer really can be beaten. You've read my story. You know there's nothing super human about me. I'm not any different than you are. Not braver, nor smarter, nor healthier, or luckier, richer or poorer than you are. I'm no more loved by God than anyone else is. I'm just me...and you are just you. And, being you is plenty good enough.

Beat the life out of your cancer, and then tell anyone who will listen how you did it. Help them out of their desperation and back to a healthy body and mind. Give them a dose of hope that only you will be able to give them. You aren't too sick, or tired, or broken...or anything. Let your courage rage against cancer. Let God show you His love.

I pray that you will find your super-human strength so you can win the battle. You <u>can</u> be the winner. I pray that you are given a monstrous amounts courage to keep you going until you're well again. I know you can find that strength. I pray that your faith grows to unimaginable heights. God will give it to you. You're alive...live and love like you're ALIVE! And, from the bottom of my heart, I wish you well.

---

### Procedure

**NM PET SKULL BASE TO MID-THIGH**

Elaine Hulliberger

---

**Final, Reviewed**
Diagnosis:
Ordered by Tania M LeBaron, MD on 2/14/2008 (Routine)
Performed on 2/13/2008 1:02 PM
Reviewed by Tania M LeBaron, MD on 2/15/2008

---

Comments: See Note (Reason For Exam
colon cancer

RADIOLOGY REPORT:
EXAM: PET SCAN SKULL BASE TO MID-THIGH
CLINICAL HISTORY: Colorectal cancer. Restaging.
COMPARISON: 02/21/07.
RADIOPHARMACEUTICAL: 12.21 mCi F18-FDG IV.
SERUM GLUCOSE: 99 micrograms per deciliter.
PROCESSING: Imaging from skull base to mid thighs with reconstructions in sagittal, coronal, and axial projections with 3D MIP images. Attenuation and non-attenuation corrected images were submitted.

FINDINGS: No pathologic areas of hypermetabolic activity were seen in the area examined. Study was normal in appearance.

IMPRESSION:

Normal study with no pathologic areas of hypermetabolic activity

Signature Line
*************FINAL REPORT***************
Read by:     Klegman DO, Steven P  02/14/2008 14:10
Released by:   Klegman DO, Steven P  02/14/2008 15:14
Transcribed by:  KSG 02/14/2008 14:15

TECHNICAL COMMENTS:
ISOTOPE: fdg, DOSE: 12.21mci, Glucose, ug/dl 99

## PET Scan

MUNSON HEALTHCARE

JFORM 4101 (7/07)

Dear *Elaine Hulliberger*        Date: 2/13/08

We wish to report the following on your mammography examination. A report will be sent to your referring physician or other health care provider.

☐ **Normal/Negative.** No evidence of cancer. If you or your doctor have noticed an abnormality such as a breast lump it is important you check back with your doctor to see if you still need additional tests.

☑ **Benign (not cancer).** If you or your doctor have noticed an abnormality such as a breast lump it is important you check back with your doctor to see if you still need additional tests.

☐ **Probably benign (not cancer).** Recommend repeat mammogram in 6 months. Please note your next mammogram needs to be done at _____

☐ **Additional imaging studies** are needed to complete evaluation, such as ultrasound or additional mammography views.

☐ **Previous films needed.** There is a finding on your mammogram that needs to be compared to previous mammograms.

☐ **Abnormal.** There is a finding on your mammogram that requires further tests for a more thorough evaluation. You should contact your physician or other health care provider within the next 2 - 3 days (if you have not already done so). Please be sure your doctor has completed your breast examination.

Interpreting Radiologist:

☐ R.M. Cover, M.D.          ☐ J.C. Johnson, M.D.       ☐ L.N. Richmond, MD
☐ D.J. Crowe, M.D.          ☐ S.P. Klegman, D.O.       ☐ T.C. Space, M.D.
☐ S.C. Hodges, M.D.         ☑ C. David Phelps, M.D.    ☐ C. J. Weitz, M.D.
☐ Ryan M. Holmes, M.D.      ☐ L.J. Priest, M.D.        ☐ T.E. Wilson, M.D.

### American Cancer Society Guidelines for Mammography

* Annual Breast Examination by a physician or other health care provider
* Annual Mammography Screening beginning at age 40
* Monthly Breast Self-Examination
* Mammography every six months for one year after lumpectomy on affected side.

Should you develop a lump or any changes in your breast before your next screening mammogram, contact your physician or other health care provider for an exam without delay.
If you have any questions please call 1-866-443-0797.

## Mammogram and Ultra sound

| Patient: | Elaine Hulliberger | Ordered: | 2/11/2008 11:16 AM by April L Moggo |
|---|---|---|---|
| Patient Id: | 156200 | Collected: | 2/11/2008 10:18 AM |
| Patient DOB: | 3/13/1943 (Female) | Reported: | 2/12/2008 7:41 AM |
| | | Reviewed: | 2/12/2008 8:24 AM by Tania M LeBaron, MD |

| Diagnosis: | COLON CANCER (153.9) | Site: | LAB |
|---|---|---|---|
| Order Name: | CA 125 | Requisition: | 0020681 |
| Status: | Reviewed | Accession: | AH9602910 |

**Result Note:**
PATIENT HAS AN APPOINTMENT 2/5/08

| Test Name | Result | Units | Normal Range | Status |
|---|---|---|---|---|
| CA 125 | **5** | U/mL | < 21 | Reviewed |

THIS TEST WAS PERFORMED USING THE SIEMENS (DPC) CHEMILUMINESCENT METHOD. VALUES OBTAINED FROM DIFFERENT ASSAY METHODS CANNOT BE USED INTERCHANGEABLY. CA 125 LEVELS, REGARDLESS OF VALUE, SHOULD NOT BE INTERPRETED AS ABSOLUTE EVIDENCE OF THE PRESENCE OR ABSENCE OF DISEASE.

# CEA 125 and Blood Work

# Epilog

We can speculate all day long about whether a doctor is getting kickbacks from the pharmaceutical companies for distributing their personal brand of medications. Maybe they do, I have no way of really knowing that. That isn't the issue though. The point is this.

If I've been told by the very people who concoct these medications that, if I take them, I could very well be the one who will end up suffering from the side effects of the drug... and I took them anyway...whose to blame for my decisions? Well, that would be me.

Take the medications that were developed to lower cholesterol for instance. I was put on them at one time. Of course, according to the advertisements on television, I should have had a blood test to see if my body would accept the drug. I wasn't given the test, and I didn't challenge the missing test. My legs began aching five days into the treatment. The doctor told me to stop taking the medicine immediately. He tried a second pill, then a third... still with no testing. I couldn't take any of them without having them affect me in unfavorable ways. So, I found a fruit based dietary fiber supplement to try. It brought my cholesterol down 30 points that put my cholesterol level well within the normal range.

If I lived in a high crime area it would be prudent to keep my doors locked, and I would. No one would fault me for that. But, if I choose to inform myself about what I allow to be put in my body, well then I'm usually viewed as a trouble-maker challenging my doctor's advice.

Challenge has very little to do with it. Troublemaking has even less to do with it. It's my body after all, and I should have complete knowledge of the medications that are being prescribed, and I should have a say, a choice, in whether I should take it or not. Truthfully, I shouldn't be put in the position of having to challenge advice from a doctor in the first place.

Let's jump from Cholesterol medications to Chemotherapy drugs for a second here. I am totally aware that chemotherapy drugs can, and do, really hurt you. I'm also very aware that without them my cancer would have put me in my grave. Without scaring the pants off of me, my Detroit doctor gave me a pretty meticulous overview of what the drugs could or would do. After that, it was my decision whether I would go on with the treatments or not. I was given the assurance that he would help me through the effects as best he could. I took his advice, and am glad I did. But, he informed me about what I was getting into and what was bound to happen to me without the drugs. I can live with that. And, as it turns out…I did. Knowing what I know now though, I would have stopped the chemotherapy drugs after I was sure it had stunted caner's growth. Hindsight is always nice. Not real productive…but nice.

As a side note here, I don't believe for a moment that cancer can't be literally cured in a more humane way. And, I don't believe for a moment that cancer isn't *very* big busi-ness. But, when you're faced with a disease that is on its way to killing you, you'll take what is offered, as it is the only hope that is available that the doctors may be aware of. That's too bad for those of us who are ill, and for those of us who are paying the bills. But, until the whole system is shaken to its core there seems to be no better answer for some of us.

## Just Thinking...

So, now I'm just thinking... What if treating cancer on an annual basis cost this country lots of money...say...in the billions or trillions of dollars? And, what if someone came along with a way to cure cancer, and the costs were... say...$60.00 or so a month? I wonder what the pharmaceutical companies, cancer researchers, lawyers, Food and Drug Administration, etc. would think? I wonder what they would do. Hummm...

I wonder what would happen if, all of a sudden, the oil cartel lost their grotesque profits because someone came up with a way to run our world on renewable, cost efficient energy? I'm thinking it would cause a bit of a stir. I think that wars are fought and lots of people die because powerful people want control over the oil reserves.

I *know* lots of people are dying on a daily basis due to cancer. And, I know what a non-toxic supplement like Protocel® has done for me, and people like me. Don't you find it curious that I wasn't told about Protocel® by the very people who are supposed to know all there is to know about the disease? Doesn't it make you wonder why the healing power of Protocel, and products and procedures like Protocel®, aren't literally splashed all over the news? Isn't it intriguing? Humm. Like I said...just thinking!

Live, my friend.

# News Paper Account

## Marion woman's seven terminal cancers miraculously cured

By Mardi Suhs, Cadillac News

MARION — At first glance, Elaine Hulliberger doesn't look like a fighter. She can't weigh more than 100 pounds and she has an easy-going manner.

When first diagnosed with cancer in 2005, she quietly followed doctor's orders.

She went home to die.

She had her best suit cleaned to wear in the casket.

Still grieving the death of her husband, who died at her feet of a sudden heart attack three months earlier, she made plans for her own funeral.

Three oncologists and a surgeon confirmed her fate and offered no treatment.

"I had cancer pretty much everywhere," she said, naming them off like an alphabet of doom — colon, liver, kidneys, bone, lymph nodes, blood, and a tumor by her aorta.

Seeing her despair, downstate family members urged Elaine to try the Karmanos Cancer Institute in Detroit.

A doctor there confirmed her diagnosis.

"He told me I was going to die but said he could give me a little more time."

That speck of hope transformed Elaine into a ferocious warrior ready to battle for her life. Angry with doctors who gave her no hope, she was determined to prove them wrong.

Two years later she is cancer free. She underwent chemotherapy and radiation at Karmanos and then journeyed to New York City to try a new form of radiation. And thrown into the mix, she started taking a dietary supplement called Protocel® that a cousin told her about.

"I didn't have anybody to talk to about it," she said of the alternative treatment. "I was alone and I was dying. Finally, I thought, what could happen? I'm going to die anyway."

She started taking Protocel and before her next round of chemo, lab work showed her blood count was up — it was normal.

Soon she was driving herself back and forth to Detroit for her chemotherapy. She was gaining strength.

She refused a second round of chemo and opted to try a new form of radiation offered at the Cabrini Medical Center in New York City.

"They chose the three areas that were most likely to kill me," she explained. "The tumor by my aorta and the tumors in my colon and liver. The doctor felt if he could give me some help with those three it would lengthen my life. But he agreed with everyone else and told me I would never get rid of this cancer."

After 11 treatments in New York, she came home last September with a CAT scan that showed she still had her tumors.

She decided that was enough treatment.

"I put myself in God's hands and kept taking Protocel."

In January an MRI showed the liver cancer was gone.

After a PET scan, her physician in Reed City, Dr. John Dennis made a startling claim: "You are not dying anymore."

All of her cancers had disappeared except for the tumor in her colon. They decided to have it surgically removed by Dr. Khatchadour Hamamdjian in Detroit.

While doing the surgery Dr. Hamamdjian took a look at her liver.

"He came to see me in the hospital," she recalled. "He said that in 25 years he had never seen anything like this — not only was my liver clear of cancer but it was healthy."

After closing down her business for two years while she battled cancer, Elaine has reopened her shop, Woodland Embroidery and Design in Marion.

She believes her miraculous cure was the result of the combination of all her treatments and her faith in God.

Now that she has her life back, her purpose and passion is to give hope to those diagnosed with terminal cancer.

"I'm not saying everybody can be saved," she acknowledged. "But you don't know until you fight and you have got to fight with every ounce of strength you have."

Elaine said she doesn't know why God spared her life. But now she intends to use that life to "help those with cancer."

news@cadillacnews.com I 775-NEWS (6397)

# Testimonies: Survival, and Caregiver's Stories

## Dennis Rogers:
## Metastatic Malignant Melanoma

I found out that I had Metastatic Malignant Melanoma cancer in 2004. I started taking Protocel 50 sometime in 2005. I was told I wouldn't see 2008 if I didn't try the Doctors drugs. In 11/16/06 I had a pet scan done here is some of what was said. "The lesions seen in the right supraclavicular area appeared to have resolved or nearly resolved. A prior small lesion seen in the left axilla is no longer present." At that time I put the Protocel 50 down because I though the cancer was gone. On 06/21/07 I had another PET scan done. The cancer came back plus it spread to some new areas. So I am back on Protocel 50.

**Dennis Rogers**

## A.M. Grover: (Florida) Colon cancer:First part of his story

March 4, 2007

To whom it may concern:
    In March, 2006 I was not feeling well and ended up in the hospital. I underwent many tests and was diagnosed with hepatitis C, cirrhosis and colon cancer that had spread to my liver.
    I had a colon resection and began chemotherapy. I began taking Protocel formula 50 on June 25, 2006. In October, I asked the doctor to retest me for hepatitis C. The result was that I no longer had hepatitis C. It was gone. The doctor told me four times that day that I did not have it because I couldn't believe him.
    I am still taking Protocel and still hoping that this will make a difference, and will get rid of my cancer.

Sincerely,
**Wallace E. Grover**

## A.M.Grover: (Florida) Colon cancer/Avastin: End of their story

    My husband, Wally, was diagnosed with colon cancer that had metastasized to his liver and he had tumors blocking his bile ducts. Wally had surgery and they removed the tumor from his colon, but the doctors were unable to remove the cancer from his bile duct. He began chemotherapy and was taking a drug called Avastin with the chemo. We discovered Protocel and Wally started taking it also.
    We really though that everything was working great together. He was able to skip the chemo and he still continued to improve. Wally's doctor continued to recommend Avastin and Wally was getting it about every three weeks.

Unfortunately, Avastin made the tumors "necrotic" (localized death of living tissue). We will never know for sure, but I wish he had not taken any of the chemicals and just taken the Protocel. The tumors were blocking the ducts from draining, and killed him. I feel as if the Avastin prevented the Protocel from working.

It is really hard to put all of your faith into one thing and really trust that it will work. I wish we had done just that.

Sincerely, Mrs. Wallace Grover

## KC: MONO
## Florida

Sam is sixteen years old. Diagnosed with a VERY bad sinus infection then five days later mono. Her white blood count was very low, her spleen very large. She was put on a steroid for three days. She was sleeping 22 hours a day not eating or drinking, she lost 12 of her 119 lbs!! After the steroid was done we tried Protocel. In just six days she was up and running around all day into the night. NOT tired at night, not sleeping in the morning!! We brought her back to the doctor her spleen was back to normal, She was fully recovered!! Praise be to God... and his protocel.

## Sara M. Sweimgon: Lung cancer

Just a few years ago I first heard of Protocel from a friend discussing it with my daughter. I didn't pay too much attention at the time, but in 2003 I was diagnosed as having lung cancer. After having x-rays and a PET scan, I decided to try it. After I received instructions on dosage etc. I began taking Protocel formula 50 four times daily, every 5 to 51/2 hours. I began taking it on July 29, 2003.

I continued this routine for 11 1/2 months at which time I had three sets of x-rays with the following results.

First set of x-rays after beginning Protocel in July of 2003:

- First X-ray: September 2003.
  o No change, tumor still showing.
- Second X-ray: November 2003.
  o Tumor still there, but smaller.
- Third X-ray: (can't remember month) 2004.
  o X-ray clear – No tumor
- Forth X-ray: March 2005.
  o Last X-ray – Clear of cancer.

While taking Protocel 50 I had no ill effects of any kind, and also had no colds of any kind and felt really good and energetic.

## Baxter the Dog: Cancer
## Owner: Cathleen Oushakoff

Baxter, a 14-year-old West Highland white terrier, was diagnosed with TCC (transitional cell carcinoma) in the bladder on Sept. 23, 2005. The vet gave him roughly 120 days to live. There was an option of chemo but without proven results. Another option was for a strong non-steroidal anti-inflammatory, which seemed to help many dogs with TCC. We decided to start on the NSAID, Peroxicam, but not wanting to give in to the disease, or leave it up to the drug mfgrs, I took Baxter to see a holistic vet. He suggested Protocel 23 and told me that many dogs live a year beyond their diagnosis. We started Baxter on that as well as the Peroxicam. After awhile the Peroxicam started causing some intestinal problems and landed Baxter back in the hospital. I had stopped the Protocel at that time too because I didn't want to aggravate his tummy with more meds. That next day, Kathie (She collects medical records from Protocel users) called and I told her what was happening and that we had stopped the Protocel. She suggested we stick with it and I agreed to try again. Well, almost 2 years have passed now since Baxter was diagnosed. Thanks to Protocel 23 he is still alive and very, very well. His cancer has not been eliminated but his doctors are all baffled by the extremely slow growth rate of the tumor. TCC is usually extremely aggressive and goes into the prostate and kidneys within that first 120 days after diagnosis. Baxter's kidneys are still free from cancer but his prostate has indeed (unfortunately) enlarged and is most likely affected by the TCC. I am convinced that the Protocel has kept the cancer from growing as fast as it would have otherwise. Throughout other bouts with stomach upset and bladder infections, I have stopped the Protocel temporarily on such occasions because again, I didn't want to bombard him with too much medication at any one time, and let's face it. Protocel tastes nasty! Perhaps if I had been more consistent with it during the more difficult days Baxter would be cancer free at this point. But I really can't complain...he is 2 years into his disease and you wouldn't know he was sick. He is as cute and loveable as ever. I am so grateful to Kathie and to Protocel for all the extra time with Baxter. He is by far the best dog I have ever had and I can't even think of being without him. Protocel is truly a gift from God.

## Joe's Story, and a Blessing from God Gail Nevitt's Caregiver's story: Lung Cancer
### Williamsburg, PA.

My husband owns and operates his own truck. In April of 2005 he was delivering a load in New Jersey and walked between two trailers to check his load. Someone had left a strap sticking out from under one of the trailer tires. His foot got tangled in the strap and he fell against the bumper of the trailer, breaking three ribs. The store manager took him to a clinic where they took x-rays and he continued his trip home.

Several days after he was home our son invited us for a cookout where he was camping. I'm not sure if it was the smoke from the fire (I prefer to think it was the Lord) but he had a coughing spell. When we arrived home that evening he was short of breath. Being the alarmist that I am, I convinced him to go to the emergency room of our local hospital. After having a scan the doctor came out and told us that we should see our family doctor because the scan showed nodules on his lungs. That was the beginning of my worst nightmare.

We called our family doctor first thing in the morning and went to his office. When we arrived his nurse came into the waiting room and said that we were to go straight to a lung specialist. We took the scan to his office and with his impeccable bedside manners, he said that he was 99% sure it was cancer. He sent Joe to the hospital for an MRI and a biopsy. We returned to his office for the results. True to form he came into the examining room exclaiming, "I knew I was right". His need to expound on his accuracy in diagnosis left me with the greatest urge to punch him in the mouth, but since my stomach was lying on the floor, I just sat there. He told us that Joe had about 4 months to live and needed to see an Oncologist and he was going to make an appointment. We informed him that we were going to go home and talk about it. After reinforcing this he still insisted on making an appointment so I told him to "do whatever" and we left. I guess he made an appointment.

I am a 24 hour hyper-activist, so I started to research and make phone calls to find out all I could about this disease and the help available. I found that Sloan Kettering in New York was rated second in the United States for Cancer. I called for an appointment late one afternoon and was told that someone would call. When no one called the following morning by 9AM, I called them. I was told that it would be at least 24 hours before they would get back to me.

I forgot to mention that along with being hyperactive I have very little patience. I called a friend and she prayed with me asking God for direction. When we were done talking I immediately called John Hopkins Hospital for an appointment. While waiting on the phone, a call came through from Sloan Kettering with an appointment. This happened one hour after I was told it would take 24 hours. God is so good!

We drove to the oncology department at their hospital in New Jersey. The doctor there said that the large nodule in the upper left lobe needed to be removed and he did not believe that the small ones in the lower right were cancer. He made an appointment with the surgeon in New York. We then went to see the surgeon, Dr Downey and he told us that he wanted to do surgery on the lower right to make sure the small nodules were not cancer because if he removed the upper left lobe and later found out the small ones were cancer we would have a real problem. We made the appointment for surgery for 2 weeks later.

I came from a suburb of Detroit but have lived in a small town in Pennsylvania for the past 30 years, so the idea of being in Manhattan on my own was a little overwhelming. I contacted the American Cancer Society to find out if there was any economical housing. They told me about a place called Miracle House. They allow patients and their caregivers to stay in a 44 floor, high-rise apartment building for a small fee. A deal considering, hotels in New York start at $200.00. A friend graciously agreed to make the trip with us. We bought train tickets (there is no parking) and the three of us left for New York. Joe had his surgery the following day. After the surgery the doctor and social worker met with us. We were told that it was cancer in the lower right and there was nothing more they could do. We were again told that he had about four months and possibly a few more with chemotherapy. I know God gave me peace (with me that's a challenge) because instead of operating in the Ozone, my feet, for the most part, stayed on the ground. For example, I'm the one who shoved my 6-week-old son at my mother telling her I had killed him, while he was screaming, because I had fallen with him. Can you begin to get the picture? Joe is not in for an easy ride! Calm is not in my dictionary.

After returning to New York for a follow up, we returned home and I began a search for the best place to receive chemotherapy. We decided on the University of Pittsburgh Medical Center in Windber, Pa. Our daughter went with us for the initial appointment. The procedure was explained to us and Joe was scheduled to have Chemotherapy for two weeks with two weeks off. I do not remember now how long the treatments were to last. I really can't tell you how I felt except to say it was like being numb. Now starts the beginning of the end. We asked both doctors at Sloan Kettering and UPMC if chemotherapy would kill the cancer. Both told us that it would not; it would only put it in remission. At some time it would return in the same place or mutate to another place. I remember saying "Lord, I really need you now!" All my thoughts were of being alone, how I would go on? Lord can we both go?

At this point I need to tell you that Joe was on prayer lists all over the country. Loving, Christian friends had phoned friends and relatives everywhere for prayer. Our three pastors had anointed him and our dear friend Pastor Pepper said he knew Joe would be okay. People never failed to tell us how they were praying for him.

We had no more than arrived home from UPMC when the phone rang. A very godly couple from our former church said "Gail get a pencil and paper, I have a word for you from the Lord". She told me how her and her husband had been praying for Joe and that weekend friends from Maryland came to visit. They told them about their son-in-law who had cancer in the bone, lung, and lymph nodes. His prostrate count was 1000. He decided to take a natural supplement called Protocel® and is now cancer free! They knew God had sent their friends from Maryland that exact weekend in answer to their prayers. I can only tell you that as far as I was concerned God had sent our answer. I knew them to be real prayer warriors and I knew God sent His answer through them. For me it was a done deal but this was not my decision.

Joe and I talked and prayed, we asked friends to pray and he made the decision to only take Protocel®. I like to say, "he "made the decision, you know, with my passive personality. This decision required a lot of determination because our family felt he needed to take chemotherapy, but the decision was made and we were on a new course, to live!

The following day I made more phone calls. I made calls to the couple in Maryland, Dr. Bell, and the company that handles Protocel®. We ordered the Protocel® and Joe started taking it four times a day around the clock. We cancelled his appointment at UPMC and made an appointment with our family doctor. Our doctor is a Christian and understood when we told him about" the word from the Lord'. We asked him to take Joe's complete care over and we would no longer be seeing other doctors. He said if we were comfortable with that, he was.

It is now 2 ½ years later and Joe is still here. We serve an awesome God!!!!! The survival rate for lung cancer is almost zero and there are usually no signs. When you finally find out it is too late. We knew someone in Michigan who was diagnosed and two weeks later died. We know it was no accident that Joe had broken ribs and had a coughing spell. A loving, compassionate, all knowing God brought them about. We have felt compelled to tell our story to anyone who will listen.

You don't have to accept the death sentence most doctors will give you, there is an answer! A loving God allowed us to receive this miracle and we have an obligation to spread the word "Cancer need not be a death sentence".

The story still hasn't ended, as God was still not through blessing me. He renewed a relationship with my cousin in Michigan who I had lost contact with for years. Her father and my mother were brother and sister. I was blessed to see her win her battle with cancer. It has been such a joy to share and be there for each other. She just happens to be the author of this book. A dear friend who was diagnosed with breast cancer is on Protocel® and doing fine. This is just the beginning!!!!

## Angela Ellis: Breast Cancer Williamsburg, PA

In October of 2006 I went for a mammogram and they discovered a small nodule. I then had an ultrasound, which confirmed the mammogram finding. An appointment was made with a surgeon. The surgeon examined me but could not feel the nodule. He wanted me to have a biopsy. I did not believe they would find cancer. He sent me to the local hospital for a scan-guided biopsy. The biopsy was performed and I was told that it was cancer and needed to be removed. This news was very unsettling because I have enjoyed excellent health and felt fine. The surgery was performed promptly and the diagnosis that it was cancer confirmed. I am a widow, my husband passed away when he was only 38 years with a heart attack. I have five children; the youngest was only 1 1/2 years old at the time. I raised my children, who are now grown and married, without the help of a father. My children were very upset at the news. Because I had not seen an oncologist for the surgery, my daughter who is an

Occupational Therapist with a master degree, insisted that I see an Oncologist it Pittsburgh, Pa. The doctor in Pittsburgh assured us that everything had been handled properly.

The surgeon who performed the surgery wanted me to have radiation. At that time I did not believe radiation to be a problem so I had the treatments. I have a friend who was given 4 months to live and did not take any treatments. He went on Protocel, and several years later is doing fine. Because of this I decided to go on Protocel myself. I have been on Protocel since first being diagnosed with cancer and plan to continue taking it. Since this happened I have done some research and learned, according to doctors, that chemo and radiation cause cancer and does not kill it. It causes cancer to go into remission and at sometime it will return in the same place or mutate to another place. If this had happened today instead of then, I would not take any treatment and go on Protocel. I have faith that the Protocel has erased the cancer. Further tests show there is no cancer.

Sincerely,
**Angela Ellis**
**Williamsburg, Pennsylvania**
**Georgeanna Rassie: Brain Tumor**

I was first diagnosed with a brain tumor in November of 1994. I had surgery after four days of steroid therapy to shrink the tumor (reduce the swelling). The tumor was 6x7 cm, and was located in the left forebrain area. Surgery removed this area in the center of the tumor to 3x2 cm. The tumor was diagnosed as a large cell lymphoma (B-CELL). This was followed by chemotherapy (systemic treatment) for approximately four months; being treated for a week and then recovering for three weeks.

After the last systemic treatment at University Hospital Ireland Cancer Center, we were treated at the Cleveland

Clinic for the BBBD procedure. The BBBD procedure is a process where a catheter is run up in the artery to the C-6 vertebrae in which a 5% mannose solution is used to shrink the blood/brain barrier membrane. Then the chemotherapy drug is introduced to the brain at a much higher concentration than the systemic was. The tumor was gone during this therapy, but came back after the second month. A different chemical was used, but the tumor still grew.

The first chemical was Methotrexate and the second chemical was carboplatin. We then went to the oral drug Temindor. At that time I was introduced to Protocel®. I began taking the Protocel® with the Temidor. I was also taking a vitamin supplement at that time. The tumor again came back.

I was informed that the vitamins I was taking was way too strong in vitamins C and E, which made the cancer cells resistant to Protocel®. So, I stopped taking the vitamin supplements and increased my dosage of Protocel® to 1/3 teaspoon, and shortened the time between doses to four hours instead of six hours.

The tumor is gone, and remains so for the past seven months. My last MRI proved that. I have been clear of cancer for the past seven months.

I am still taking the Protocel®, but will stop for three months, then go back on it for three months. I feel as though six months of taking Protocel® is a long enough time because I am post cancer free.

I have had no ill effects from taking the Protocel®, but the chemotherapy treatments really did beat up my body physically and mentally. The cancer was only in my brain, but is now gone.

I did do other things to help my body's immune system, such as juicing and drank and ate only chemical and hormone free organically raised foods.

Sincerely, Georgeanna Rassie

## Mary Huchins: Bladder cancer

To Whom It May Concern:

In August of 1997 my urologist told me that I had an adenoma carcinoma of the bladder. I then had a test of the colon, which was negative for cancer.

Over the years my bladder was checked periodically, and new sites of cancer were removed. Finally, in April of 2005 the cancer had spread to the urethra. My urologist told me to have the bladder removed. I declined his recommendation for a less drastic treatment. I started taking Protocel® four times a day on June 26, 2005. Both of my physicians checked me at the hospital, and everything was clear.

Later, a PET scan was taken, and the diagnosis was 'unremarkable'! I continue to take Protocel® everyday.

Thomas Schwahm: Kidney cancer

I was diagnosed with kidney cancer in 1997. The urologist explained the only treatment was to remove the affected organ. Sometime later I decided to have elective surgery for BBPH. The routine X-ray showed the cancer metastased to my abdomen and lung. In my travels I met a lady from Ohio who was taking what she called 'Cancell', and she suggested I start taking it immediately for my returned cancer, (the name has changed to Protocel®), and I started in 1999 and have taken it ever since.

The records show I was cancer free in 2001, and I still am. Because the only cancer treatment I was doing for this period was taking Protocel®. There is no other reason to believe it not cure my cancer.

Sincerely,
**Thomas Schwahm**
**Ruth Keller: Lung cancer Cadillac, MI**

I am Ruth Keller. I live in Cadillac, MI. I was a healthy 66-year-old woman until, in April of 2006, I got pneumonia with a large mass on my lungs. A month later, after X-rays and a biopsy, the doctor discovered I had non-small cell lung cancer.

I June I heard about Protocel® from my sister-in-law who has a business in Cadillac, MI. There was a lady that had come into her business and shared her story about how she had cancer throughout her body and took Protocel®, and was doing great!

I told my sister-in-law to order the Protocel® and the book, *Outsmart Your Cancer*, on the Internet.

I took the Protocel® before my surgery. After the surgery the doctor said I might have to have chemotherapy. When I got home from the hospital I started taking the Protocel®. It made the pain much more bearable, and I seemed to get much stronger.

I realize that God had led me to the Protocel® and that He is the healer of all diseases.

When I went to the cancer doctor in September of 2006, they were amazed how good I looked and how well I was doing physically. I told her that I was taking Protocel® and the Protocel® vitamins.

In December of 2006 I saw a different cancer doctor from Grand Rapids, MI. He said I was doing so well that he did not need to see me until July 3, 2007. That will be one year after my surgery!

I am so thankful to God for finding out about Protocel® and I give Him the glory!!

**Sincerely, Ruth Keller**

# My Life Beyond Cancer: Alan D. Johns – Prostrate Cancer

My name is Alan Johns, a retired naval aviator, 75, who should be a prime candidate for prostate cancer. In my diagnosis in 2005, an invasive (through the colon wall) biopsy was used. I was alarmed, but had put my care (and life) into the hands of a local urologist, who performed this procedure himself on an outpatient basis at the rural (but magnificently business-like) hospital. He gave me a few antibiotics, but I came down with septicemia, for which I was rushed to the ER and was admitted with "pneumonia" in mid summer by my alarmed wife.

If I exhibit some disdain for the medical profession, it is because of that botched biopsy.

That urologist diagnosed me with prostate cancer with a cancer- marking blood test (PSA) at 11.7. My sister had been introduced to a website, "outsmartyourcancer.com" I already had read articles skeptical of cancer treatment as a moneymaking endeavor of doctors. I was interested not in continual treatment, but a cure. I went to the recommended website, WebND.com and ordered 1 quart of the mixture called "Protocel® 23". The "23" formula was intended for the "milder" cancers. It's intent had to be disguised as "dietary supplement." My sister also told my life-long smoking brother about "Protocel® 50." He took this, extending his life a year until he died of emphysema at age 64. I believe he was cured of lung cancer.

In my prostate cancer case, I changed physicians because I wanted relief from the urinary symptoms of an enlarged prostate. He recommended the Tran urethral resection, commonly called the "roto-rooter." I underwent that in a three-day stay at an urban hospital. Tissue reamed from my prostate exhibited cancerous cells at a Gleason scale "9."

This urologist left the "natural means" treatment up to me; so, I resumed five daily doses of Protocel® 23.

I see this urologist every six months because the last PSA was 2.73. The previous bout with prostate cancer brought my PSA down from 11.7 to 2.5. The previous urologist was impressed, saying, "A man of your age should be about 6."

I continue on a maintenance dose of Protocel®, which costs about $133 for a two-month supply (with shipping clear across the country from N.C.) The routine-change in my life now entails carrying a "kit" with a glass and a plastic bottle with a pre-measured dose and a bottle of distilled water. I wake at 3:00 A.M. to use that kit in the bathroom where I have ceased to need to go. I feel grateful to be on a maintenance schedule till my next six-monthly blood test.

I recommend Protocel® to all my friends. One, I was not prompted to tell just died of pancreatic cancer; of which he died in the same month he was diagnosed. People who have a history of cancer in their families should use it as a precaution. Protocel® 23 is this world's best anti-oxidant. That may explain how it starves cancers for oxygen. My schedule is ¼ tsp in 8 oz of distilled water at 8:00 AM, 1:00 P.M, 5:00 PM, 10:00 P.M. then (after setting an alarm) at 3:00 A.M.

I wish you all as productive a life as I am having after cancer (and before).

## Cancer is a Challenge

**By Ken Browne**
**Queensland, Australia**

Cancer is not just another challenge in life - but a challenge "For Life". So we need to plan wisely and in most cases quickly.

We have another problem in as much as what each of [our] bodies are willing to accept. What works for me - will not necessarily work for you.

I am new to this disease, having only been diagnosed on 10th May 2006 and I started taking Entelev, which is the Australian name for Protocel®, on 19th July. I have been taking it for around one month now. And my health has improved so much I am no longer taking prescription drugs for my blood pressure, cholesterol and many other health problems. A hand full of pills that used to start my every day has been reduced to just one!

I would like to share with you some things that my wife and I have found out about how to be confident in our approach to fighting my cancer, which is in the pancreas at Stage 4, mass in my liver, stomach arteries and ten other legions as per my C.T. Scan diagnosis.

When we received the news about my cancer we were like everyone else. The first week we had to console each other - sometimes when just thinking of the cancer tears would well up in both our eyes. It was then that we decided to think positive and formulate our "Fighting Plan".

The Oncologist did not even want to know me and told my doctor over the phone "Tell Ken to come and see me when he cannot stand the pain any longer". Consequently I have had no conventional medical treatment whatsoever!

I continued to visit my own doctor of 15 years once a fortnight to get my blood pressure checked and for vitamin B12 injections. He is now totally amazed at my present health, as three months ago he gave me six months to live.

In the beginning I mentioned that everybody's "body" is different. As in most cases we all have other health problems to contend with. Mine is having had a number of strokes which left me a disabled pensioner at 50 (now 70). My Warfarin (a blood thinner) medication has to be kept stable so as not to cause me to have another stroke.

We started with a Naturopath who refused to consider my overall general health requirements. Needless to say we now have $1000 of supplements stored in a cupboard that we may never use. We soon found this to be a very expensive exercise; brought about by rushing into something we knew absolutely nothing about.

She did however share some very important things that needed to be addressed immediately. Like to detoxify my body and change my diet to a raw green leafy vegetable one. Detoxifying my body believe me was one experience that I could have done without, as sitting on the toilet all night just did not excite me in winter time.

Looking back though I believe it did my body a lot of good, as from then on I started to shed the extra weight that I was carrying and I lost around one and a half kilos per week on this diet without even trying (from 110 kilos to 87 kilos in just three months). The reason for the body detox is that our body stores toxins in our body fat and this is just another "Body Product" that cancers can feed on.

Added to this she recommended - no dairy products, no red meat, no white bread or flour, no processed foods of any kind or foods with preservatives added, no soft drinks or alcohol and definitely no sugars or any fats, no fruits that are full of sugar such as bananas and watermelon. All fast foods were definitely a real NO-NO!

She also told us where to buy apricot kernels and to said to take about 30 a day, but what she didn't tell us was that our body processes these in about 80 minutes, and that they needed to be taken in regular hourly doses. So you see there are many things that you have to find out for yourself.

One very important factor that we have in our favour is by being on the Internet we have many more opportunities than other people, as we were are not totally bound to what conventional medicine dictates for us.

After buying the book "Out Smart Your Cancer" and progressing to Entelev/Protocel® we were able to read about other people's cancer testimonials, and now have no doubt whatsoever that we will be one of the "Winners" in beating my cancer.

We have found the main things to do are:

1. Initially, you have to move quickly away from "Why me, or Oh poor me". Think positive and be confident that you will outsmart your cancer.
2. You need all the support you can get from your spouse, neighbour, or a good friend. Don't suffer in silence but be careful of people who want to give you negative input as this can only lead to more stress and you don't need it. It's your body and you need to keep your head positive in order to survive.
3. Constantly take it to the Lord in Prayer! I tend to always pray like our "Saviour did on His cross, Loving heavenly Father if it be possible let this Cup pass from Me"! But not My Will, "Thine Will be Done", always ending with please "Bless those people that are also praying for me."
4. I would go for the detox as we also found the weight loss beneficial, along with a diet that you feel your body is most happy with. You can be sure that it will tell you this. I still have two meals a day with raw green leafy veggies on them. For breakfast I have a soft-boiled egg with them for my protein and for a drink I have ginger in lemon juice. For my mid-day meal I alternate fish (salmon) and chicken. My drink is most times orange juice freshly squeezed. For dinner (as it is winter here in Queensland Australia) I like chicken veggie soup that my wife makes for me. As a drink I have chamomile herbal tea. A small amount of fruit is added to all meals as a side dish. For supper I

have Bio-Dynamic Yogurt (no fat) and strawberries to keep my bowels happy. Beverages are made up with two liters of tank water daily, herbal teas and freshly squeezed orange juice. I tried to drink raw veggie juice but my body reacted with vomiting. Added to the above we always endeavour to purchase organic products and we grow all of our own vegetables.

5. My Lysing. I have found to date that it consists of a rash to my upper body and gas in my bowel. We put the small amount of lysing down to having had the earlier detox!

6. If you decided to start on Entelev/Protocel® make sure you read the instructions on the bottle and stick to the recommended dose. Taking more only costs you money and taking less at intermittent times is life threatening! The manufacturers have designed their product for the maximum impact on you cancer so it is advisable to follow their instructions to the letter. With regard to the times to be taken - it is every six hours.

We did not want to sit up to midnight every night for years so I set the alarm for 4am and I start to take the first one then - so this means 4am, 10am, 4pm and 10pm, which also suits us better for taking on an empty stomach. We have two small 40ml bottles so that we can premix my medication and we also take these with us when we travel. I fill one of these at 10pm so as I am prepared my 4am medication before I go to bed at 10pm. We also take our own tank water with us when we know we are going to be away at my medication time, as it has no chemicals added. The manufacturers say to take one quarter of a teaspoon and as we did not get a measure when we purchased our Entelev we have worked it out as 19 drops per 150 mls of water. I like to measure it out into a 20 ml medicine glass with water added, then drink it down, followed by drinking the further 150 mls.

7. With regards to the supplement Entelev Proteolytic Enzymes capsules, I take these three times a day at 9am, 3pm and 9 pm, again on an empty stomach.

I decided not to have another CT Scan until I finish the first bottle of Entelev in another two months time.

Another suggestion I would like to make is that when you have a CT scan and they measure it, ask them to do a density test on the cancer to see if it is shrinking from the inside.

We hope that everyone will be encouraged to continue to "Fight the good Fight"!

## Cheers and best wishes to all from Carmel and Ken in Queensland, Australia. We have an opinion.

People today have been brain washed into believing that doctors are the only ones who have the answers. We will never be able to correct that fallacy until the conventional medical community recognizes the truth about natural treatments as a valid alternative and/or partner to harsh drugs. We have been told that it is unethical, even unlawful, for conventional doctors to recommend or advise the use of natural, alternative medicines. Medical schools don't teach their students about natural supplements, and I wonder why? I wonder who supports the medical universities in this country? It could be the drug companies... If that's the case, their own agenda, which could be driven by dollar signs, may have a great deal to do with their lack of enthusiasm where drug-free, alternative medicine is concerned. Don't you think? Patients are convinced that doctors, pills, and potions are the quick fix for everything. However, pills and potions are a cure for nearly nothing, especially cancer. If you have a rash, been in an automobile accident, or have broken a bone, then doctors are who you want to deal with. Otherwise, it is prudent to shop around.

There are a lot of people who believe it is the cancer patient who has been denied treatment from their doctor who has the best chance of survival from terminal cancer. The ones who the doctors won't treat because they feel there is no hope for the patient. That is when the survival instinct gets in the driver's seat. Survival is the strongest natural instinct in every living thing. It was my own survival instinct that cleared my head and brought me to an agreement with Protocel®. The time has come when it is necessary to take control of our own diseases and look at alternative methods, and remedies. It doesn't cost you a dime to look at alternative medicines, but it could cost you your life if you don't.

People, these days, can build their own homes without the help of professional builders. They paint their own homes without painters. They sell their own homes without real estate agents. They can defend themselves in courts without lawyers. They can learn all about what is going on in the world with the help of their Computers. Organic farmers are still growing their crops the same way that their fore fathers have done for centuries, and with excellent results. As you can see I have spoken of the D.I.Y. (Do it Yourself) world we live in. As you know, many people have had bad experiences with the trades-persons above. Some professional people have ripped us off, as well. So, you get the gist of what I'm trying to convey. If you can't trust them, then D.I.Y. However, with trades-people or professionals, our life isn't on the line. When a doctor rips you off, or makes a mistake, you may not be around long enough to get angry about it.

Why then are many doctors still being treated like they are the all-knowing Gods?

Then why, do we do exactly as they tell us without question? It is because we have total faith in them? Or, isn't it closer to the truth that we've all just been conditioned to believe that we can't survive without their conventional treatments? Have doctors ever ridiculed you because you believe in natural supplements? I'll be you have. Natural supplements work, so do you ever wonder why they do that?

A thing we must remember is, doctors are medical practitioners. 'Practitioners' indicates to me that they are "Practicing Medicine"? If that is difficult for you to read and believe, then think about how many diseases can actually be cured. Even the common cold eludes the medical community. I can't cure the common cold either, but I can alleviate it's symptoms more humanely with natural supplements than they can with medication that can/will cause a whole host of other maladies that are far worse than a simple cold. How many times have we sat in a Doctor's Office and listened to them say that the medication they 'tried' on you is not working? Don't they want to try (practice) with another medication? Each person is unique. No one drug works for everyone. When it's your body that the side effects will cause harm to, what do you do then? In addition, what will they prescribe to alleviate the side effects? After that, what can they offer you for your original health problem? It can, and often does, become a vicious circle and your heath can be the payment for their experiments. How many people with cancer have had their Chemotherapy changed for the same reason? Have you even been a witness to a patient whose first chemotherapy treatment has nearly killed them? I have. It's all so scary, isn't it? Do you think some doctors may need more practice, and aren't you the one that will be practiced on? There was a case that we witnessed here in Bundaberg Australia a couple of years ago. Many people died, or were maimed for life, as the results of a bad surgeon. Do you think he should be excused because he was just" practicing"?

Alternative medicines have been used here long before there were any universities where doctors could study and learn their craft! The Chinese have used ancient herbs and medical methods to cure people since the Middle Ages. "Years teach more than Books" It was GOD who put all the minerals, herbs and spices on this earth.

They were put here so as we could make ourselves healthy by using them as everyone had to do in the EARLY DAYS!!!

PLEASE don't get us wrong we fully Recognize and give Credit to the Brilliance and Dedication of all the Doctors, Scientists and Pharmacists, plus the people who made it their life's work to Perfect and Produce Alternative Natural Methods of Medicine that can cure many Diseases. Much of their work was (and still is) constantly hampered by Politics and the large Pharmaceutical Companies who want to make billions from our sufferings by pedaling disease medications that in some cases do not work!

Our greatest need today is to build our own bodies Immune System Up with a Proper Natural Diet, so that it can fight all of our diseases from within! Not bombard it with Foreign Chemicals from without that it cannot handle. Many of these Chemicals damage the Good Guys as well as the Bad Guys!

Natural Dietary Supplements created from God's STOREHOUSE of minerals, herbs and spices, used correctly will treat the complaint CAUSE for a SUCCESSFUL RESULT.

NOT just the SYMPTOMS as some Pharmaceuticals Companies Medications DO!!!

Your Life is your Own—Take Control!

## Charlie Meese: Prostrate Cancer
## Pennsylvania

When attending a doctor's visit in August of 2006 for uncontrollable urine, I was diagnosed with a urinary tract infection. The blood results also showed a PSA of 16.00. I was also told that I had prostrate cancer.

In that same time frame, I also heard of Protocel®, I started taking Protocel® on September 13th, 2006. Within then next three months and after another blood test, my PSA was 3.2.

Having had several eye operations in the past eight (8) months, and having to have blood work done before an operation, my PSA has remained stable to this day. My success can only be attributed to Protocel®.

Sincerely,
Charlie Meese

# Websites and books

Don't be afraid of cancer. Inform yourself, then, get on with your cure. You'll find a wealth of information that these people have complied for cancer victims. Victims…just like you and me.

**Ty Bollinger:** *Cancer: Step Outside the Box*
http://www.cancertruth.net
Mr. Bollinger has written one of the most comprehensive books on all the aspects of cancer that I have ever read. If you're looking for inspiration, answers, hope, courage, and faith: run…don't walk to his website and purchase his book. You will finally have the insight on the business of cancer that you couldn't find anywhere else. Amazing!

**Tanya Harter Pierce: Outsmart Your Cancer**
www.outsmartyourcancer.com
In Ms. Pierce's book you'll find a ton of information on cancer and alternative treatments to help you in your fight against cancer. You can purchase her book on her website.

### Pamela Hoeppner: The Breast Stays Put
http://www.thebreaststaysput.com

Pamela Hoeppner has written a superb book about her battle with breast cancer. Her book is available on her website, and is packed with insight, humor, and answers to questions that you'll need to get you through your own personal nightmare of breast cancer. She truly is a joy to read, and a real inspiration.

Http://www.elonnamckibben.com:

Mrs. McKibben has a tremendous cancer survival story that inspired me to keep my fight with cancer going strong. She is an amazing woman. Her testimony is one that kept my courage and faith strong so I could whip the disease. It's worth your time. Take a look.

### Kathie: kathiedub@aol.com (Director of medical record collections for Protocel®)

Kathie will encourage you, and help you with answers where she can. She is a good person to have on your team.

www.altcancer.com
www.protocelforum.com
http://www.cellremoval.com
http://webnd.com
Where you can purchase Protocel®
**(866-766-8623)**
http://www.Protocel Golbal.com

http://www.altcamcer.com
http://www.protocelglobal.com
http://www.protocelforum.com

## Where to buy Protocel:

**Vitamin Depot**
330-634-0008
www.yourvitamindepot.com

## Renewal & Wellness
http://www.webnd.com
866-766-8623